MAKING MIRACLES

MAKING MIRACLES

FINDING MEANING IN LIFE'S CHAOS

Paul Pearsall, Ph.D.

AVON BOOKS ◆ NEW YORK

The ideas, procedures, and suggestions contained in this book are not intended to replace the services of a trained health professional. All matters regarding your health require medical supervision. You should consult your physician before adopting the procedures in this book. Any application of the treatments set forth in this book is at the reader's discretion.

AVON BOOKS
A division of
The Hearst Corporation
1350 Avenue of the Americas
New York, New York 10019

The Prentice Hall Press edition contains the following Library of Congress Cataloging in Publication Data:

Pearsall, Paul.
  Making miracles / Paul Pearsall.
    p.   cm.
Includes bibliographical references and index.
  1. Pearsall, Paul—Health.   2. Cancer—Patients—United States—Bibliography.
3. Miracles   4. Prayer   5. Alternative medicine.
I. Title.
RC265.6.P43A3   1991
362.1'96994—dc20
[B]
                                                                    90-29011
                                                                    CIP

First Avon Books Trade Printing: January 1993

*For everyone who prayed for me, especially my wife, Celest;
my sons Scott and Roger; my mother, Carol; my brother,
Dennis; and the spirit of my father, Frank.
Thank you for my miracle.*

ACKNOWLEDGMENTS

Book acknowledgments often begin with the sentence "this book would not have been possible without the help of . . ." In the case of *Making Miracles, I* would not have been possible without the help, energy, prayers, and support of hundreds of people who made the miracle of saving my life. My wife, Celest, is the most powerful healer and miracle maker I know, and I owe the fact that I survived almost certain death to her love, sacrifice, and enduring faith. Her love for me is a miracle. My son Scott showed unimaginable courage and caring through my crisis, and he is one of the bravest persons I know. My son Roger gave me energy and could send his love from anywhere at any time. My mother, Carol, lost my father, Frank, much too soon, and her heroism in the face of also almost losing her son gave me comfort in my pain and helped me feel the presence of my father's spirit. My brother, Dennis, was always there to help. This book is not only dedicated to my family but is a direct result of what I learned from their collective ability to make miracles.

There are too many healthcare professionals to name who were also miracle makers. Dr. Robert Bloom never doubted the power of his craft, and his clinical nurse, Marilyn, was always patient with my fear. Dr. Lyle Sensenbrenner, Dr. Joseph Uberti, Dr. Voravit Ratanath, and all the doctors of the Bone Marrow Transplant Team at Harper Hospital in the Detroit Medical Center literally saved my life. I will never forget them and I hope this book will bring others to them for the magic of healing. My nurses, including Chris, Pat,

Carolyn, Marjorie, Betsy, Andrew, Maryann, and Rosie, were my true life-support system.

The original and pioneering work of Dr. Larry Dossey was the primary influence that drew my attention to the new physics behind miracles. The writing of physicist Dr. Harold Morowitz, who shares my love affair with the island of Maui as a symbol of the wonder and joy of the forces of nature, provided clarification regarding the necessity of local pain for the privilege of cosmic joy. The other great scientists whose work and ideas are described in the following pages provided the material to help me understand the miracle of life.

My agent, Susan Cohen, stayed with me through my suffering and encouraged me to write this book. My editor, Toni Sciarra, helped me to say what I felt and shared her personal wonder at the feelings and facts behind miracle making. Finally I want to thank my hundreds of co-authors, patients like Patsy who suffered along side me on the bone marrow transplant unit. We did it! We made miracles! This book and my living would not have been possible without all of you.

Paul Pearsall, Ph.D.
Maui, Hawaii
December 25, 1990

CONTENTS

Each self is a divine creation.
—SIR JOHN ECCLES

MAKING MIRACLES

1

MIRACLES, MAUI, AND ME

A Postcard from Paradise

I'm not afraid of dying. I just don't want to be there when it happens.

—Woody Allen

To the Magic Kingdom or the Science Center?

I died. I'm back. I was near death three times, but I am writing to you from my home in the paradise of the Hawaiian island of Maui from where I hope to share with you my celebration of my several miracles and my discovery that miracles do not "happen." I know now that miracles are *made*, and this book will teach you how to make your own miracles in your life and the lives of your loved ones. We can make these miracles by combining the principles of modern science with faith in the boundless capacity of the human spirit to discover a deeper logic and meaning in the life crises, the strange coincidences, and what frequently appears to be the total chaos of our daily life.

I have been a researcher, author, and hopeful skeptic all of my adult life. During my formative years as a scientist, two of my visits made a lasting impression on me. More than a decade ago, I lectured on the campus of UCLA. As I entered the physics build-

1

ing, I saw these words of the meticulous experimenter Michael Faraday carved in stone just over the main entrance: "Nothing Is Too Wonderful to Be True." The book you are about to read will document that you do not have to accept bizarre beliefs about astral projection, hauntings, channeling, psychic energy, or the Bermuda Triangle to discover as I did that every aspect of our own existence is miraculous.[1] You will see that within our very nature is a wonderful and wondrous capacity to create the miraculous.

My second significant visit took place a few years ago. My family and I flew to Orlando, Florida, to visit Walt Disney World. As we left the airport grounds, we saw the pair of road signs that are still there. They require a quick decision as tourists rush through their busy lives. One sign reads "This Way to the Magic Kingdom" and points toward an enchanted place called Walt Disney World. The other sign reads "This Way to Reality" and points toward the Space Center at Cape Kennedy. We decided then to make the time and effort to go to both places, and I invite you to take the time and make the effort to visit both the world of dreams and the world of science as you travel with me through the merging point of these two realms.

The glitter and thrill of our fantasies and senses are easy and fun, and they are well worth the trip. Although less accessible and requiring more intellectual effort, the world of science also holds its excitement and titillation, but more patience is required. *Miracles are made when these two worlds combine.* If you feel confused or overwhelmed by a scientific principle presented in this book, remember the two signs in Orlando. Remember that we are used to traveling in only one world, the world of what we have come to call reality. Few of us will become astronauts and experience firsthand what the reality of science can accomplish, but if you are willing to learn how to travel through both the worlds of science and spirit, you will discover that anyone can become a "miracle-naut."

If you become confused, keep reading. Further examples and clarification will follow. The first part of this book is the most difficult because it introduces complex scientific principles that, although they have shaken the very foundations of the scientific community, have gone largely ignored by the general public. The principles of science are less seductive and immediately intense than the ride on Space Mountain in Walt Disney World, but they are no less thrilling and much more significant and enduring. The miracles that result from the merging of science and spirit will become clear through the true stories and scientific studies found here. These accounts and precepts are wonderful, but they are not too wonderful to be true.

I will show you that *we can all be miracle makers because we are at the center of the universe where science and spirit meet.* Each of us represents the merging of these two systems of explaining life. Author and pioneer in the study of human consciousness John White writes that the view that we are the center of the universe is not meant egocentrically or astrophysically but rather as a "point of confluence for higher and lower worlds, the visible and the invisible, the mundane and the sublime."[2] Where science and spirit meet is where miracles explode into being.

A Vital Voyage and a Study of Miracle Makers

The pages of this book describe my own journey through the intense reality of excruciating pain, illness, and near death, to the heights of magic and mysteries of my cure that can be understood only from the point of view of a parallel world of dreams and miracles. I will describe my survival of two "terminal" cancers, the near-complete destruction and regeneration of my bones, three surgeries, two drastic chemotherapies, massive whole-body radiation, a bone marrow transplant, near-fatal pneumonia, serious threats to the health and lives of my family, several near-death experiences, and remarkable coincidences that occurred throughout this vital voyage. All of these events took place in less than one year that seemed sometimes like a decade and at other times like moments.

I will also describe the science behind the facts of levitation, traveling through time, seeing without looking with the eyes, altering the past, remote viewing, sharing consciousness with animals and plants, miracle healings, the power of prayer, and research findings on the right and wrong and effective and ineffective way to pray. I report on findings from my twenty-year study of seventeen miracle makers. Through my years of practice, I collected data on seventeen patients who, according to traditional medicine, were dying. All of these people were miracle makers and came to call themselves the "MMs." All patients were seen by me in the Problems of Daily Living Clinic in the Department of Psychiatry at Sinai Hospital, in Detroit, between 1972 and 1988. Each patient was given a verdict of "terminal," which they converted to a diagnosis of being in a state of "dysmiracolia" or in need of the making of miracles. They showed courage and an uncommon consciousness. I am now preparing a detailed report on the diseases, treatments, and miracles of each of these patients. I include their testimonies along with my own as evidence of miracle making derived from our own involuntary, chaotic experiments in the development of our souls. These experiences became the crucible in which a new blend of rational and spiritual concepts was formed. The result is my recipe for miracles.

A Place to Become More Alive

I am writing this book, and live much of my life, in Maui, Hawaii. Mark Twain visited Maui and wrote, "I just got back from the beautiful island of Maui. It was the most sublime spectacle I had ever seen. I think that I shall remember it always."[3] Maui symbolizes the confluence of the natural wonders of science and the mystery of what Hawaiians call *aloha*, or "loving spirit." Native Hawaiians say *Maui no ka oi*, which means "Maui is the best," and the remarkable weather, beaches, plants, and people blend in a joyful jubilee that substantiates that claim. I have always come to Maui to write my books and to bask in the *aloha* and *koomohalu* ("love" and "relaxation") of this paradise. When I began to die, however, I learned that Maui was much more than a place of magnificent beauty. Through its formation, mythologies, and legends, Maui is a symbol and metaphor of our potential as miracle makers. In this and in later chapters, I will use Maui's rich spiritual tradition and natural beauty to clarify the concepts of miracle making.

My gardener, Pete, was born and has lived his life in the paradise of Maui. When I returned to Maui to heal, Pete sat with me under our monkeypod tree. The sprawling branches of this tree spread like a huge umbrella to filter the sun into tiny sparkles that danced on our faces. "Maui is a different place," said Pete. "In Maui, you become a little more alive every day. In many other places, unless you try very hard, you seem to die a little every day." This book is about "trying very hard" by learning the basic principles of a newly emerging science that can help us tap our innate capacity as miracle makers.

Combining *four general theories* and *six specific scientific principles* derived from the startling new cosmic and quantum science, I will share *ten sacred secrets of science* for the making of miracles. Each is revealed in the magic of Maui that Mark Twain felt. It is the same magic that helped me to heal. I have been literally within seconds of death. I have felt what it is like to be a ghost. I have felt the power we all have to be akin to Maui, the demi-god who used the power of his spirit combined with the natural wonders of the world to fashion the miracles of Maui from the eruptions from the sea, just as we can make miracles from the turbulence of the chaos of our lives.

Maui was half-man and half-god. He pushed up the sky so people could rise and walk. He caught and tamed the sun to create time. It is likely that he is a deified Hawaiian ancestor of great strength and wisdom who actually lived in the islands. Although he is the favorite god of Hawaiian mythology, he is not worshiped. Like all miracle makers, he is seen as the common man extended to remarkable limits. He was a Polynesian prankster: an ordinary person who combined the traits of Hercules and Paul Bunyan to become an adventurer, trickster, and maker of real miracles. In his ability to span both the physical and spiritual worlds as half-man, half-god, Maui embodies our own potential to merge science and spirit in making miracles.

The chapters that follow will uncover the ten secrets of science that offer explanations for one or more aspects of miracle making. As this book progresses, these principles will be combined to form the template for the construction of your own miracles.

We Aren't Here, We're Everywhere

The *first* general theory of new science to be described is that of *nonlocality,* or the fact that people and events can "happen" instantaneously everywhere, anywhere, and at any time. Nonlocality means that because we are all a part of God we are all everywhere and a part of everything. We are a body and a brain, but we are also a part of, influence, and are influenced by the stars, the sky, and one another. Like Maui himself, each of us is godlike and personlike because we are each a manifestation of God's presence in everything. This means that we lead a divine life even as we lead our daily life. Maui helped to create his world, and as philosopher Ernst Lehrs points out, "The path of all . . . leads from being a creation of God to becoming co-creator with Him."[4] We make our miracles when we discover the godlike characteristics in ourselves that transcend our here-and-now bodies. Author John White writes, "At the heart of all things . . . is a spark, an impulse, a sense of the Divine."[5] Miracle making is a common human trait that grows from this spark of divinity shared by all of us. As Maui sparked his island to life, so we energize our lives and those with whom we live. It is not the achievement of supergurus and a select, lucky few that accounts for miracles: It is the fact of our godlike essence and our freedom from a local body and place-restricted view of self.

Believing Is Seeing

The myths of Hawaii teach that the Hawaiian Islands were created by Maui and his brothers pulling the islands from the sea. Maui warned his brothers that if they looked back as they pulled, their observations would cause the large land mass they were tugging on to remain partially under water. The brothers chose to see things their way and stopped to observe what was happening. As a result, instead of one large mass in the middle of the Pacific, dozens of islands stick up as punctuations for each pause to peek taken by the Maui brothers.

The *second* general theory from new science is *observer partici-pantcy*. Like the Maui brothers, scientists profoundly determine what is discovered by the act of experimentation. Researchers know that what they discover is profoundly influenced by what it is that they are looking for and how, when, and with what they are doing the looking. Replication (repeated studies) and double-blind experiments through which the scientist and the subject both are unaware of what is being studied are two attempts to control the powerful influence of the observer creating the results of the experiment.

You will see in a later chapter that the act of observation actually physically alters the nature of what is being observed. Whether or not scientists see a particle or wave of energy is determined by what they choose to look for and what they choose to look with. If they look with a particle detector, for example, a particle will occur and they will see a particle. If they look with an energy detector, a wave of energy will occur and they will see energy. As unbelievable as it may seem, we see what we look for and create what we see by how we see. Our reality is created from the act of our own observations.

Because of our capacity to create our reality, it sometimes seems as if we were watching ourselves live in the form of a spiritual instant replay. You may be aware of a time when, just as you were closing your car door, you noticed your keys still in the ignition. You may have said to yourself, "There are my keys that I am about to lock in my car." You shut the door and curse your helplessness as you stare at the keys. You knew you were going to do it. You saw yourself doing it before you did it. You got what you were seeing, but perhaps if you had been looking for a different vignette, the keys would be in your hand rather than dangling defiantly inside your car.

A blob of ink on a white card is an arrangement of ink particles or a butterfly, depending on who is doing the looking. A basket of fruit is the source of a snack or a potential work of art depending on whether or not a hungry person or skilled artist is the viewer. Beyond mere interpretation, observer participantcy teaches us that we create our own reality by our point of view. Just as the observer creates what is observed, we make miracles by *choosing a miraculous view* of our lives.

With Uncertainty, There Is Always Hope

Mythology aside, the islands of Hawaii were created by a land mass moving architectonically over a hot spot on the ocean floor. As the mass moved over that spot, immense explosions shot the land to the surface of the sea, creating the 130 islands, islets, and shoals that make up the Hawaiian archipelago. Through the centuries to this very moment, eruption of the volcanoes of Hawaii continues the birthing of the islands.

Haleakala volcano, a mass of lava rising 30,000 feet from the ocean floor, where my house is located, is still situated on the hot spot. There is constant uncertainty as to when the next eruption of lava might occur. The more we feel we know the island as it is, the less we know of what it could become. The *third* general theory of new science, the *uncertainty principle*, suggests that this same uncertainty applies to all of our lives. You cannot identify one event or aspect of your own life that is totally and absolutely certain. Even the nature and meaning of our death and what may follow it remains a matter of speculation unclarified by the medical reality of the death and dispersing of the personal pile of molecules we use as a vehicle for our "self." The chaos we see every day is evidence of the constant state of flux that characterizes the universe. All life is an undetermined work in progress.

The one sentence I use most often with patients who are suffering from a deadly illness is "In the absence of certainty, there is always hope." If you or someone you love is ill now, remember that not one doctor can be entirely certain about the course of the illness. Doctors are shocked daily by the fallibility of certainty. The doctors who help us make our miracles recognize and acknowledge their uncertainty to their patients. By helping us remember this uncertainty, they guarantee our hope.

The Hawaiian Islands reflect this uncertainty. They are constantly changing, so no one can be certain if their home is built securely and forever on a lovely, peaceful beach or sitting in the path of a tidal wave or volcanic flow. Like our entire life, it is precisely this threatening but dynamic nature of the islands that results in the eternal optimism of the native islanders, who have learned that ultimate beauty always arises from the most turbulent times. Constant change and chaos guarantee the validity of hope, because eternal change means that anything is possible.

There is, however, one exception to the uncertainty principle that I will discuss later in this book. We can be certain of the fact that relationships never end. No matter how angry, hurt, or afraid we become, we forever share our spirit with those with whom we become close. I suggest that the human spirit—our shared and infinite (nonlocal) oneness with each other—resides temporarily within the physical body but forever within our relationships. We are eternally the sons and daughters of our parents, the wives and husbands of our spouses, the parents of our children, and the students of our teachers. Death changes but never ends these relationships. There *is* one certainty in the world: Relationships are everlasting.

Look At Life from Both Sides Now

Haleakala volcano last erupted about 200 years ago. It is massive, young, and potentially volatile. The west Maui mountains were formed by the extinct volcano Puu Kukui. It is 2 million years old, twice as old as Haleakala. Maui is old and young at the same time, and one cannot fully understand the nature of this beautiful place without knowing both the legends and the newness of the island. There are opposites to everything in the universe, and miracles are made *when we remember to draw our strength from a holographic or complete view of life rather than a one-sided image.* Old and new, particle and wave, hot and cold, and love and hate always exist simultaneously. We view the world with only one eye when we neglect the complementary side of any issue in our lives.

This holographic view of life is summarized by the *fourth* general theory of new science, the *complementarity principle.* Research has shown that the "quantum stuff" of which all of life is made is simultaneously both wave and particle. Understanding the complementary existence of these two opposing states (energy and mass) frees us from creating artificial boundaries between the body (mass) and the spirit (energy). This freedom makes any miracle possible. Our miracle point of view (observer participantcy) sets the stage, our shared faith and hope (nonlocality and the uncertainty principle) furnish the energy, and the knowledge that existence is not singular or one-sided (complementarity principle) supplies the raw materials for our miracle making.

We're All Number One

Maui is called the Valley Isle because the east and west Maui mountains, with their differing histories and myths, are joined by a sprawling isthmus or valley. Likewise, our world civilization has been characterized by a tenuous connection between the Western world's reliance on facts and technological progress and rationalized religious belief and the Eastern world's orientation toward faith, a sense of timelessness, spiritual evolution, and a more metaphorical and philosophical spiritual view.

This tenuous East-West connection exemplifies a *fifth* scientific principle. This is the concept of *oneness,* or the fact that everything in the cosmos is inseparable. The closely related principle of non-locality defines our shared and timeless omnipresence within the universe, and the oneness concept emphasizes our connection with one another. I will describe how the "strange" coincidences that often erupt in our lives are actually surprise clues that can help us reconcile and connect the spiritual and rational worlds and rediscover our oneness.

In order to build a bridge like the valley between east and west Maui, miracle makers learn to *combine* the Western world's "profane" or here-and-now emphasis on being objective, doing, succeeding, and exerting technological control with the more "sacred" Eastern world orientation of equanimity, subjectivism, balance, acceptance, and riding with the universe instead of trying to drive it. *Miracle makers draw from both East and West to find a center from which their miracles can emanate.*

The Levels of Life

The *sixth* finding of science teaches that there are several *levels of reality* including but transcending our local see-and-touch world. The *kahunas,* ancient "spiritual leaders" of Maui—who practiced the *Huna* secrets of spiritual healing—defined illness and personal crisis as becoming trapped in one level of reality and saw ultimate healing as restoring a person's ability to know and experience all levels of the reality of their spirit.

As an objective scientist taught to search for one true reality, it was difficult for me when my own near-death experiences forced me to confront the fact that there exist many domains of reality and that each realm had its own unique rules. My own miracles, and the miracles of the seventeen miracle makers whom I studied, have exposed realms of reality I never could have imagined. Miracle makers cross easily between these realms and are not blinded by the glare of the common consciousness required to survive from day to day in the sometimes overwhelming see-and-touch world.

Time Doesn't Tick

The demi-god Maui was able to alter time. He fashioned a rope and lassoed the sun as he stood on Haleakala. In other words, Maui knew how to create his own time. I have found that this same skill applies to all miracle makers.

My house is *makai,* or "toward the ocean" from the Haleakala crater, in a subdivision called *Hale Lakau,* or "house of the setting sun." It is one of the few places in Hawaii where sunrise and sunset can be seen clearly from the same spot. I can feel the *seventh* secret of science: the principle of *relative timelessness.* Every day, as I sit on my *lanai* ("porch") and watch every white-yellow sunrise and every golden-orange sunset, I sense the circularity and relativity of time. Each sunset seems to be the prelude to the next sunrise and each sunrise seems to be an invitation to take part in the passage to night. Creating miracles requires that we free ourselves from the profanity of linear, man-made time and, like the demi-god Maui, claim our own elective, sacred time of celebration of every moment free of ticking clocks.

University of Oxford physicist Roger Penrose writes, "The future and the past seem physically to be on a completely equal footing. Newton's laws, Hamilton's equations, Maxwell's equations, Einstein's general relativity, Dirac's equation, the Schrodinger equation—all remain effectively unaltered if we reverse the direction of time."[6] It did not take "time" for Mozart to compose his complex masterpieces. Mozart writes that his work "did not come to me successively . . . but in its entirety." Mozart saw his entire symphonic work "at a glance."[7] Our most creative scientists typically describe their miracle discoveries as taking place when they freed themselves from the mechanical measures of directional time. Creative people characterize their work as spontaneous, co-incidental, sudden, and even surprising. This has been called the "Aha! phenomenon." Our coincidences and our miracles seem characterized by this same spontaneity and timelessness. Miracles are made when we learn to be free of a linear time line and understand that past, present, and future are not separate.

The Ultimate Paranormal Event

The *eighth* secret of science is the existence of *growth energy fields* that influence the development of all living things. The seventeen miracle makers whom I studied were acutely aware of the impact of these energy fields and were able to use and direct them in their miracle making. *Sudden coincidences are the pulls and pushes from these growth energy templates.* We can discover the potency of these energy fields by paying attention to and reflecting on every seemingly serendipitous event in our life.

   Human life is the ultimate paranormal event. What makes us live? Where does our life energy go when we die? The science concept of growth energy fields provides insight into the immortality of life energy. Miracle makers know that there is a "fifth force" or a spiritual energy that exists beyond the vague concept of "psychic energy." There are more than 100 names for this "fifth energy" found in cultures throughout the world, including the Christian concept of the Holy Spirit, the Chinese concept of *chi*, and the Taoist term *qi*. On Maui, the ancient healers use the Polynesian word *mana* to represent the energy of the spirit. Just as scientists once doubted how an invisible gravitational force emanating from the moon could affect the ebb and flow of the tides on earth, so science traditionally has been reluctant to study the fifth energy. Now, however, scientists have begun to study the fifth energy by discovering some of its consistent characteristics.[8] Among its many characteristics is that it is not weakened by distance (nonlocality); it is seen more easily by some observers than others (observer participantcy); it has its exact opposite form of energy, which is negative and disruptive (complementarity principle); it is constantly ebbing and flowing and changing its strength and impact (uncertainty principle); it has a "sticky" nature that unites and combines (oneness); it is absorbed by organic material, such as humans and animals, but is refracted by inorganic material, such as metal and certain toxic materials; and it tends to concentrate at certain locations throughout the world. One of these locations is Haleakala Crater on Maui. In its secret science center at the very top of Haleakala, the U.S. Air Force is using lasers to continue demi-god Maui's pursuit of the sun and the stars. These experts have measured the various energy fields of this volcano. Its forces are immense. The healing energy from

Haleakala, as you will read later, was strong enough to whirl me around in my bed to a healing posture!

Why Does Everything Seem to Be Falling Apart?

The *ninth* science secret of miracle making is *entropy*. Derived from the Second Law of Thermodynamics, entropy is a concept that predicts that everything and everyone is in the process of falling apart and burning up. As violent as this sounds, entropy is in fact a process and not a verdict regarding our existence. Entropy is really a *positive* and necessary force that is one aspect of our movement through the chaos of living. *We are only falling apart so we can fall together again in a different and higher order.*

Making miracles requires learning how to use our crises and times of falling apart as vehicles for movement toward an ever-evolving and developing human spirit. Our crises are not evidence of our final failure to survive. Quite the contrary. Crises are evidence of our survivability and continued development. Crises are our experience of the chaos caused by the fifth energy constantly stirring things up to higher and more-developed levels. Miracle makers have learned not to complain about the size or taste of their piece of the world pie. They are busy enjoying and helping to make an entirely new pie.

The island of Maui still has small earthquakes almost every week as Haleakala quivers in anticipation of further growth. *Tsunamis*, or "tidal waves," still occur, as well as hurricanes and floods. Like everything in our universe, Maui is still in chaos, going through entropy, falling apart. The result is a magnificently evolving miracle: a constantly emerging and dynamic new paradise.

Miracles are maps through the chaos. In fact, miracles, like Maui, are possible only in the presence of entropy and chaos. Without chaos, life itself and the miracles of living would not be possible.

A New View of Order

The *tenth*, and final, science secret is the new field of *chaology*, or the study of chaos. Science has discovered a remarkable, stunning order within chaos. Making miracles requires the skill of seeking and appreciating the "chaotic order" that is a natural part of our existence. Like miracle makers, scientists are learning to celebrate rather than fear chaos and to look within it rather than away from it for clues to the meaning of our living. Like the air we breathe, chaos keeps us alive.

Climbing the Path to Haleakala

When you climb Haleakala, the difficulty of the journey sometimes distracts you from seeing the overall beauty of this magnificent place. The large ferns and tropical plants seem chaotically scattered in your way. There is, however, always another turn in the path and the beauty of the magnificent crator draws you upward. The farther you go, the more the majesty of your voyage becomes clear and you begin to feel a part of the crater itself. As you journey through this book, have patience and trust that the beauty of the making of miracles will carry you through. If you seem to miss a point along the way, it doesn't matter. Keep going. You will come to that point again. Your spirit knows the way.

In the next four chapters I present in detail the first four sacred secrets of science as they relate to miracles. These are the four basic principles of nonlocality, observer participantcy, uncertainty, and complementarity. We will explore the meaning of coincidences in our lives and the importance that "chance occurrences" have in helping us to make miracles. I will show you how to set the stage for miracles and describe the common characteristics of the miracle makers whom I have studied. I will also describe my own miracles as an example of a scientist who rediscovered his spirit in the chaos of his own near death.

The final six chapters provide the six remaining sacred secrets of science. Each describes a specific scientific finding as it applies to the making of miracles. Each chapter presents one phase of my struggle through life-threatening illness, a bone marrow transplant, and on to a complete cure. I will take you with me through the agony and joy of dying and being reborn and the chaos of my chemotherapy, near-total wasting away of my body, radiation therapy, and the threat of a severe viral pneumonia. Together, we will discover how love embodies the sacred secrets of science that lead the way to miracles. The book concludes with a minimanual for making your own miracles.

The demi-god Maui performed the miracle of ordering chaos. He raised the sky and tamed the sun so people could stand up and walk in the dignity of their own sacred time. Maui's miracle created an island of wonderful chaos that contains nearly every geographic and climatic feature on earth. A cosmic clutter of rainbows arch everywhere through the valleys and over the lush green mountains that wear cloud leis of white and gray. The sea roars; then is silent as the trade winds howl and whisper. I can rest here in this place of miracles. I can envision the sublime spectacle of the miracles I will share in these chapters and pray that my sharing will help you create your own miracles. Through this postcard from paradise, I wish you "much love and learning in your journey," or in Hawaiian, *Aloha nui loa!*

Paul Pearsall, Ph.D.
Maui, Hawaii
August 8, 1990

NOTES

1. For a careful description of the application of sound science to "paranormal events" by some of the leading scientists of our time, see O. Abell and B. Singer, eds., *Science and the Paranormal: Probing the Existence of the Supernatural* (New York: Charles Scribner's Sons, 1981). See particularly the article by Massachusetts Institute of Technology physicist Philip Morrison, "On the Causes of Wonderful Things: A Perspective," 349–362.

2. John White, *The Meeting of Science and Spirit: The Next Dynamic Stage of Human Evolution and How We Will Attain It* (New York: Paragon, 1990), xiii. Dr. White describes the emergence of humanity to the stage of *Homo noeticus* (new state of knowing, or "noetics"; what I will call in this book an "uncommon consciousness"), or a state of new awakening to the meaning of life as a unified and shared experience with all of the universe. Just as humankind has evolved through the Neanderthal to the Cro-Magnon stages, we are now beginning to reach up (science) and divinity is beginning to reach down (the Spirit) to take us to a new awareness of our status as miracle makers. Dr. White also provides a clear description of the levels of spirituality in his essay "What Is Spirituality?" in the text mentioned above.

3. Quoted in Robert Wenkam, *Maui No Ka Oi* (Deerfield, IL: Tradewinds Publishing, 1988), 2.

4. White, 168.

5. *Ibid.*, 4.

6. The fact that the equations of physics and quantum physics have no preference for evolving in a future direction is a difficult concept to grasp, but it is scientific fact that, as Penrose points out, "The future determines the past in just the same way that the past determines the future," Roger Penrose, *The Emperor's New Mind: Concerning Computers, Minds, and the Laws of Physics* (New York: Oxford University Press, 1989), 306.

7. See Jerome Hadamard, *The Psychology of Invention in the Mathematical Field* (Princeton, NJ: Princeton University Press, 1945), 16.

8. Ivan Sanderson, "Editorial: A Fifth Force," *Pursuit* 5 (Oct. 1972). He, along with author John White, are among the first to identify and write about the characteristics of what they call the X-energy, or fifth energy.

2

BURNED CANDLES, FALLING
CLOCKS, AND GOLDEN BEETLES

The Meaning of Miraculous Coincidences

> The more absolute death seems, the more authentic life
> becomes.
>
> —JOHN FOWLES

Are Our Coincidences Coincidental?

I waited for the phone call that would tell me whether I would live
or die. Our home was quiet except for the ticking of an old clock
that had hung on the wall for more than twenty years. The doctors
suspected the worst. They would be calling any minute with the
results of a biopsy of an apparent tumor in my lower back. Our
lives seemed precariously suspended in time as my family sat with
me, staring at the phone.

With a loud crash, the old clock in the kitchen near the phone fell
to the floor and shattered. None of us moved as we looked helplessly at the scattered mess of glass and metal. Within seconds
after the crash of the clock, the phone rang. I answered the phone
and held the receiver for my family to listen with me. "I'm afraid
your time has run out" said the doctor. "The biopsy shows a

virulent cancer that has spread through your bones." Like our shattered clock, our life was left in shambles.

Throughout this chapter, I will describe how to understand the role of coincidences such as the falling clock and similar meaningful patterns of chance in providing clues to our destiny. The first clue in making sense of coincidences is to understand that *coincidences follow the principle of nonlocality:* They do not happen separately from us but rather are manifestations of our own energy.

Just because coincidences happen in the outer world does not mean that they have to remain there. We can choose to view our coincidences as what psychologist Carl Jung called "synchronicities," or bridges between the worlds of matter and mind and science and the spirit.[1]

There is no question that the dramatic chance joining of events in space and time can be explained on one level of reality by statistical probability. In the game of bridge, a hand of all hearts has a 1 in 10 billion chance of occurring, and when it happens it is truly amazing to the recipient of this apparent gift from the card gods. Scientists know, however, that any other specified hand of cards is equally unlikely to occur.[2] Most of us who do not regularly deal with mathematics and statistical probabilities tend to underestimate the frequency with which rare events do in fact occur (a 1 in 1,000 occurrence will virtually certainly occur in 10,000 trials). That such coincidences can have meaning for us cannot be dismissed by science as what some statisticians call the "gambler's fallacy." Each coincidence in your life provides you with a choice of whether or not to use that coincidence as a life lesson or to dismiss it as a statistical fluke.

Prehistoric Coincidences

One of the leading researchers of synchonicity, scientist Arthur Koestler, writes, "There exists a phenomenon . . . which has puzzled man since the dawn of mythology: the seemingly accidental meeting of two unrelated causal chains in a coincident event which appears both highly improbable and highly significant."[3] Scientists know that our finding of drama and mystery in our coincidences has evolutionary significance.[4] It has always been important and adaptive for our ancestors to look for the meaning behind the significant or coincidental events of their precarious lives. If a Cro-Magnon man or woman saw a large boulder fall loose from the wall of their cave home just when they were pondering the whereabouts of the closest beast, it was not unwise for him or her to wonder at the boulder's movement taking place just before a large hungry animal stomped by the entrance to their cave and just when they were thinking about their safety. Even if boulders are statistically due to fall loose at any time, and even if the vibrations of the tiger's steps may have freed the boulder, there has always been something adaptive in looking for the many meanings of the coincidences in our lives. Better to be impressed with our coincidences than to stumble into a beast or ignore information that can teach us about survival. Seeking the meaning of inexplicable events in our lives is an instinct and enables us to adapt, learn, and evolve.

Our *consciousness* can evolve only if we are willing to risk looking for the meaning of our lives as rigorously as we adapt to the world in which we live. Coincidences are one source for such meaning. Psychiatrist Richard M. Bucke wrote, "When we are in tune with a consciousness of the cosmos, we become members of a new species."[5] Just as Cro-Magnons advanced beyond *Homo erectus* and the Neanderthals by developing a sense of meaning, symbols, and a higher level of knowing, so we move closer to our miracle-making destiny by learning to interpret our coincidences as deeply as we analyze their statistical patterns.

Philosopher Sven G. Carlson writes, "Chaos and chance are words to describe phenomena of which we are ignorant."[6] But we do not have to remain ignorant. New science is beginning to explain the miraculous significance of the coincidences in our lives.

Moments for Miracles

"He may never come out of this," murmured the doctor to my wife. I was totally paralyzed, but I could feel every puncture and pull of the needles and tubes. I struggled to raise my eyelids, but my body was not responding. I tried to signal by twitching my wrists, which were bound to the bed to prevent me from trying to pull the breathing tube from my throat.

"Those little twitches are normal when you're dying," said a nurse to my eighteen-year-old son. He was crying, "No, no, he isn't dead. I can feel his life in there."

I thought, "After twenty-five years of my own research and writing about illness, healing, and death, is this what death really is? Do you lie for eternity, aware, but trapped in a decaying body? I'm so much more than this body, but people think my body is me. Do you hear your family crying at your funeral? Do you hear your friends saying that it is a shame that you died so young? Do you lie there in that dark coffin thinking about everything, but separated from everyone forever?"

My body seemed strangely alien to me. It was a source of pain and entrapment; a used vessel that was suffering separate from "me." I felt that my family, my friends, my mother, my father, and all of my deceased relatives were with me. I felt more connected to everyone in my life than I had ever felt before, yet I was being declared disconnected by mechanics who read the gauges measuring my body machine as being beyond repair.

I wanted to scream, "I'm alive! I'm alive! Don't let my body fool you. Don't leave me to rot. I'm still me. I'm here with you." The panic burned my eyes as my soul screamed for recognition, but no tears would come. My body would not do the crying for my spirit. "It" wouldn't cry for "me."

Suddenly, a new sensation. "I feel something. I feel raindrops on my eyelids. It's raining on my eyelids. Maybe it always rains in heaven. Are these divine drops of holy water? Maybe it's from all the clouds floating around in heaven that I had always seen in pictures. Maybe it's rain from the angels' clouds."

I felt the burning dryness of my eyes being washed away, and I heard my son and wife sobbing over my face. I felt their sobbing shaking my bed. Their tears were falling on my eyes, somehow seeping in and causing my own tears to flow.

"My God," screamed Betsy, the joyful and always-hopeful nurse whose voice had so often comforted me and whose healing energy I could always feel but whose face I had never seen. "He's crying. Those are his tears, too. Look." I felt my wife and son grab me, ignoring the crash of bottles and wires that collided around me.

"Hold him," cried my wife. "Don't let him slip away."

Seeing Better with Your Eyes Shut

I had never been able to see Betsy, but I knew exactly what she looked like. I knew that she had dark hair curled around her head and that her teeth never showed even though her smile was broad and warm. I knew how tall and how heavy she was, and I knew her caring eyes were a light blue much like the light over my bed. I knew that the first finger on her right hand had a gold band and that she often cried when she laughed. I knew that, unlike many medical health workers, she wore her stethoscope over one shoulder instead of around her neck. For Betsy, a stethoscope was a redundant piece of hardware. She was able to interpret the rhythms of the heart without artificial amplification.

My body was unable to do the seeing for me, but I saw Betsy nonetheless. I "saw" every nurse and doctor, even though I never opened my eyes before this wonderful moment. Freed by the tears of my family, my eyelids popped open. I recognized Betsy, my wife, my son, and every detail of the room I had never seen.

A miracle had been made. It was fashioned by human hope and love. It was brought to life by *the coincidence* of my wife's and son's tears falling directly into my own eyes to help them see again.

Being able to see with my physical eyes seemed unimportant, however. My experience of "seeing without looking" is substantiated in a recent report by internist Dr. Larry Dossey.[7] Dossey describes a patient undergoing surgery whose heart suddenly stopped beating. Frantic efforts by the entire surgical team managed to revive her. Once back in her hospital room, the patient reported "a clear and detailed memory of the conversation of the surgeons and nurses during her cardiac arrest."[8] She described the operating room layout to the smallest detail, the hairstyle of the scrub nurse, and even the fact that her anesthesiologist's socks were mismatched on that day.

The "Doctors' Dirty Data Dodge"

This patient's doctors, as did many of my doctors, dismissed her reports, saying that such reports are "common after crises and anesthesia." Doctors often require commonality as represented by large numbers and significant statistics in order to accept research findings, but when it comes to affairs of the soul, they view the commonality of experiences as being counterindicative of their existence.

Patient reports about miracles, meaningful coincidences, and seeing without looking are viewed by physicians as "dirty data," probably because such information contradicts their more mechanistic view of the human condition. They have mistaken the strength of their remarkable methodology for truth itself.

Quacks, Quirks, Jerks, and True Healing

Whenever I lecture about the "commonly uncommon" occurrences that take place in medicine, skeptics point out, as one doctor said to me recently, "The whole field of medicine is getting populated by just plain quacks, a few quirks in the data, and a whole bunch of jerks." We all agree that there is never an excuse for harming a patient.

However, if "experimentally proven" is the single criterion for a "nonquack" medical practice, then almost all of modern medicine is pure quackery. Less than one in five of all currently traditionally accepted medical practices has been proven effective in well-controlled, replicated studies over time. The remaining 80 percent of everything that is commonly done to us by doctors and hospitals has never been thoroughly and conclusively researched.[9] Medicine is truly an art, but it has become an art limited by its own structures, and this fact sometimes gets in the way of healing. Miracles provide as much important data as computers. Artist Pablo Picasso wrote, "Computers are useless. They can only give you answers."[10] Making miracles is the art of discovering and asking entirely new questions.

An ancient Chinese proverb says, "The bird does not sing because he has an answer; he sings because he has a song." Making miracles requires that we look with as much vigor at the melody and symbolism of individual coincidences (such as my falling clock and my wife's life-giving tears) and miracles (such as seeing without looking) as we do scores of data about hundreds of events.

Uncommon Sense

Now here's the kicker to Dr. Dossey's example of one patient's perfect vision of her medical emergency: She had been totally blind since birth! Unlike me, this woman had had long experience in seeing without looking, and her ability to see during her emergency treatment convinced her that, as Dr. Dossey writes, "Sarah now knew that the world worked differently than anyone supposed, there were principles operating beyond the common view."[11]

Yale University biophysicist Harold J. Morowitz writes, "The cosmic grandeur of the universe does not spare us from local pain."[12] He suggests that *the workings of the universe as revealed by new science also explain the miracles of our daily life*. Although it is dangerously selfish to spend our lives in cosmic wonderment and ignore the reality of pain and suffering, it is also wrong to limit our view to local, mechanical, individual experiences of pain and suffering and live in denial of the principles of cosmic joy and miracles. As Dr. Morowitz writes, "Between experiencing cosmic joy and alleviating local pain there is a path that each can follow."[13] I think I have found at least a partial start on that path, and I invite you to join me in a journey along the path to cosmic joy.

By one of the coincidences I have described, I encountered Dr. Morowitz's book about geology and mysticism in a small store in Franklin, Michigan. I was browsing for some new reading material when I noticed a book with the fascinating title *Cosmic Joy and Local Pain*. As I thumbed through the book, I saw the island of Maui on the inside cover. The book sits beside me now as I write this sentence in my home in Maui. The inside cover shows a map of Maui, which looks not unlike the image of a man gazing down to contemplate a small neighboring island. I was struck by the fact that the man seemed bent over. Even though my own pain was soon to cause me to bend in agony, I only see the significance of that coincidence in retrospect. I remember being drawn to the book by that map because I had just finished building my dream home on Maui. I had always hoped to be an author and to write my books on my *lanai*, or "porch," overlooking the ocean. There has always been something special here in Maui that brings me closer to the cosmic laws that seem so remote in other places. The same year that I completed my house and began to realize my dream, I became "terminally" ill with cancer. Now, I'm here again and writing this book.

I didn't know when I read Dr. Morowitz's book that I would soon struggle on the most personal of levels with the conflict between cosmic joy and local pain. I later applied the insights I gleaned from my coincidental encounter with his book to my experiences as a scientist and as a person who has felt the worst of local pain and the miraculous healing power of the principles of cosmic joy. As a result, I can begin to explain how the laws of the cosmos also are the laws of miracle making.

Local Suffering, Cosmic Cures, and the Principle of Nonlocality

The meaningful coincidences in our lives, seeing without looking, and understanding that there are several ways of "knowing" are evidence that there is much more to us than skin and bones and days and years. The local or here-and-now world is often characterized by suffering, grief, and pain but we are not bound by the mechanical limitations of Sir Isaac Newton's one-cause-and-one-effect world. A preliminary step in making miracles is taken when the pain of our local suffering is placed in the context of the laws that govern the universe rather than being viewed as the immediate discomfort of our local daily lives.

The experience of Dr. Dossey's patient reminded me of a deaf patient of mine who years ago wrote a note to me when she was in intensive care. She wrote, "Will you please have them turn off that infernal heart monitor buzzer. I can't sleep with that constant beeping noise." Playing my doctor role, I patronized her by pretending to turn the monitor off. I was sure that she was "just upset" and not making much sense.

Less than an hour later, the head nurse called me to say, "Your patient is really angry. She told you she couldn't sleep with the heart monitor beeping and you said you would turn it off. She fell asleep for a few minutes, but you didn't turn it off and it woke her up."

I rushed to the unit and turned the machine off. She slept soundly through the evening until another nurse on a later shift turned the beeping sound back on. The patient awoke suddenly and screamed. The nurse was startled at her deaf patient being bothered by all the noise. In that moment, she learned that there is much more to our world than mechanical explanations of the here and now.

I later apologized to my patient for my narrow and uncaring

view of what it really means to hear and sense the world around us, particularly when we are in distress. I now know from my own experience that we are more than the sum total of firing neuronal gaps. We are not just our body, and we are not just here now in time.

Nonlocality is the central assumption of quantum mechanics, a remarkable new branch of physics. These are the rules of the goings-on at the subatomic level: the laws of the very, very small going very, very fast. Quantum mechanics also clarifies the miracles that we live every day—the synchronicities and coincidences that can mean so much—and provides a framework for understanding how the principle of nonlocality exhibits itself in our lives.[14]

The principle of nonlocality holds that people and things are affected by events that are not just in the here and now. This can be a very difficult concept to accept in the common consciousness. We are raised believing that we are made up of parts, that our parts wear out, and that we die. We are taught that effect always follows cause and that our identity is limited by physical, mechanical laws. As one of my despairing patients reported, "Look. We're real for a while and then we rot. Eventually, our clock breaks or runs down and we die. Our time runs out. Life is a crap shoot." As common as these "local" assumptions about life are, they are all wrong.

In accordance with the laws of the quantum world, there are several levels to our living and knowing. The miracles and mini-revelations that take the form of significant coincidences in our lives are evidence of our nonlocality.

The Language of "Lumps" or "Jumps" and the Principle of Complementarity

Sir Isaac Newton formulated a mechanical theory of a universe that operated like a perfectly coordinated clock. The principles of miracles, however, are found within the science of new physics, relativity theory, and quantum mechanics. These principles all suggest that we are not just "stuff." According to the newest scientific laws, we are "everything."

Physicist, philosopher, and psychologist Danah Zohar writes,

"The most revolutionary, and for our purposes the most important, statement that quantum physics makes about the nature of matter, and perhaps being itself, follows from its description of the wave/particle duality."[15] This scientific principle asserts that all being can be described equally well either as particle or wave; as material or motion. We are not just "things" that eventually burn out or break. We have life on an energy or "wave" level in addition to our "particle" selves.

The complementarity principle of new science, first formulated by physicist Niels Bohr, tells us that all that *is* can be described either as a temporary freeze-form of "lumps of stuff," or as being in temporary transition through an "energy jump." When we learn this dualist and dynamic state of our existence, we are liberated from the prison of being "things in a local world."

When my cancer was first diagnosed, I remember feeling that something was wrong in my back long before I actually was diagnosed as being sick. I remember feelings of energy flowing in unusual ways in my lower back. I told my wife, "It's like someone is running electricity through my lower hips. It's like they are buzzing." By the time X rays were taken to show a soccer-ball–size lump, there were months, perhaps years, of "energy jumps" of this disease throughout my body. Just because a lump could now be felt did not mean that "energy jumps" were not still taking place, however, and I knew that if I were to fall into the "locality trap" of seeing things in mechanistic ways, I would never be able to "deenergize" my cancer. I would limit my miracle making by the local view that I "was a thing with a thing" instead of both energy and mass dancing back and forth forever.

One of the major mistakes that oncologists and their patients make is reflected in their language of locality, a "lump language" that ignores the duality of mass and energy. They speak of mass, grades of mass development, spreading of tumors, excising or burning out the mass, and shrinking the lump. The new science theory of observer participantcy teaches us that the observer becomes a part of, and in fact creates, what he or she observes. How we will experience crises in our life such as cancer is thus largely determined by our point of view, and the actual disease process itself is influenced by the impact of our observations on every cell in our body.

Messes, Miracles, and Observer Participantcy

The principle of observer participantcy reveals that the act of observing alters what is observed. Extending this idea into daily life, we either make a mess or a miracle of our own life depending on the meaning we choose to give to our living. Whether we see limited and local order in a universe of total chaos or an infinite order revealed through what appears to be chaos is, therefore, one of the key choices of our lives, because in choosing a world view we actually create the world that we experience.

Author Louise Hay writes, "Life is really very simple. What we give out, we take back."[16] Such a view has sometimes been distorted to mean that we cause our illness because of some bad thinking or feelings. Its true message, however, affirms our power not to be passive observers of our lives. We cannot ignore the seriousness of illness, but miracles are made when we remember that we are a part of and not the helpless victims of the challenges of daily living.

For example, if we choose to view AIDS passively, seeing it as being caused exclusively by an uncontrollable "thing that gets in the blood," we miss the opportunity also to deal with AIDS as energy disruption and to create the miracles that can come from the energy transfusions from friends and loved ones. If heart disease is seen as being caused by having a Type A personality, we are deceived into thinking that one irrevocable cause equals one irreversible effect. If family strife is ascribed to the latest buzzword *co-dependency,* we fail to understand our potential for repairing family life on a spiritual energy level, not just on an interactive, behavioral level. The old medical saying, "It matters less what type of disease the patient has than what type of patient has the disease" means that the observer is a participant in and partial creator of what is observed and that there are complementary sides to every aspect of our existence.

If you can see only masses, then you'll receive mass repair. Doctors will cut and burn away the unhealthy structures, but they will fail to help you dissipate and diffuse the disruptive energy also involved. This energy is the nonlocal cause of the coincidences that sometimes startle us. It is a "fifth" energy far stronger and more pervasive than gravity, electromagnetism, and strong and weak nuclear energy.

If you look only for this fifth energy, however, you will miss dealing with that transient state of "stuff" that can be vanquished by some of our machines and chemicals. If you see only psychological causes to disease, for example, you miss the complementary fact that heredity, genes, and environment are also important in understanding, preventing, and fighting illness.

One of my seventeen miracle-making patients (MMs) joked, "I'm sick of this psychological stuff. Now I'm told that my attitude made me sick. What about just plain bad luck? I'm sure the roll of the genetic dice plays a role in all of this. Do you want to know the number one cause of a problem like infertility in the United States? It's a well known fact: If your parents didn't have children, then you won't, either." Of course, you would not be here to have fertility problems if your parents never had you. This patient's point is that we sometimes get so caught up in complex psychological theory that we lose sight of the more obvious causes of our problems.

Physicists know that observation alters what is observed. In my own case, I put the principle of observer participantcy to work by choosing never to see my cancer as just a lump. Instead, I saw some of my cells as overgrowing due to contaminated energy. I knew that the complementarity principle asserted that both aspects of my cancer—both the lumps and the energy—had to be dealt with. I took the poison given to kill the lumps, but I also attempted to reenergize the healthy cells in my body and to crowd out the pathological energy. I remained aware of my cancer as both lumps and jumps. I am sure that many of my miracles were due not only to good medicine, doctors, and nurses, but also to this "dualistic imagery" based on the principle of complementarity and wave and particle duality theory. Whether the poisonous chemicals used to kill the fast-growing cancer cells in my body were caustic or curative depended in large measure as to how I chose to see them. Using the principle of observer participantcy, they would be seen as vital life-giving fluids clearing the way for the growth of healthy cells. I called my chemotherapy my "life lubricants" and "saving solvents" rather than caustic killing chemicals, and because that is what I saw, that is what they became. Through the alchemy of my perceptions, toxic medicines were converted to healing solutions. I urge anyone who is ill to remember the phrase that "what you see is what you get" is an invitation to healing, not a way of fixing blame for illness.

Overcoming the Ultimate Miracle Blocker

Guilt is the number one block to making miracles. Popular psychology wrongly and dangerously suggests that we make ourselves sick by thinking the wrong way or by being a Type A or some other letter of the alphabet, and many suffering patients and their families must endure the added burden of self-blame, guilt, and doubt. As a result, miracle making is obstructed.

"I know that I caused this cancer," sobbed the young woman. "I've read all about it. I was depressed about my divorce, so I became a Type C or a cancer-prone personality. I didn't love enough. I ended up ruining my immunity and then I got cancer."

This statement by a frightened and now guilt-ridden patient reflects the dangerously simplistic orientation that has developed in recent years concerning personality and disease. Miracle making is not a competition that leaves the losers to die. Making miracles involves seeing life *and* death in the context of the miraculous.

Some of the miracle makers described in this book were not cured, but they were healed. Their healing involved the miracle of a new holistic view of themselves, their lives, and their loving. As scientist John White writes, "Healing is not always cure. Nor does cure always involve healing. Healing pertains to the spirit, cure pertains to the body-mind." Healing refers to discovering our nonlocality and "awakening to God,"[17] or the self that lives beyond the mechanics of our bodies. In Latin *curare* means to "fix and repair." *Haelen* means to "make whole." It is when we feel one with God and are aware of the sacred principles of our nonlocality and unity that we make the miracle of healing.

The Physics of Parenting: New Science in Daily Life

In his proposal of his theory of complementarity, physicist Niels Bohr was the first to discuss how waves become particles and particles become waves depending on how they are observed. Bohr often used his own personal interactions with his children to illustrate his point. When one of his children misbehaved, Bohr found it difficult to inflict the necessary punishment. He wrote that he could not "know somebody at the same time in the light of love and in the light of justice."[18] Bohr suggested that you would be whatever you saw: a loving parent or a rational judge. Parenting fails when we try to violate this principle of complementarity by being all things to our children at the same time. Complementarity and the new physics of better parenting suggests that we choose one role best suited for one time, see ourselves clearly in that role and work hard to fill it, and then look again for other roles that may be of help.

Extending physics to parenthood may seem awkward, but when Copernicus altered our view of the earth as the center of the universe and when Newton provided his laws for tracking the movement of the stars and the planets, their discoveries altered forever the consciousness and practices of everyday people. With the remarkable findings in quantum mechanics, we have an opportunity to evolve a new consciousness. Making miracles depends on understanding the profound truth that our perceptions create our reality and that there is always another view of every issue. If we let the consciousness of new science affect our world, then things—including miracles—do not just happen *to* us; we *make* them happen. Our consciousness is not "local" or inside us. Our consciousness is nonlocal. It moves everywhere and affects everyone and everything.

Three Lessons of Healing

If you know someone who is seriously ill or in crisis, remember to tell him or her three things we have learned about miracles and healing.

First, tell such people that they did not cause their problems. Guilt is a killer, not a healer. Being sick is a necessary part of living. Emotional states and personalities are not the single direct cause of any disease or crisis. Even when we can identify the germ that causes an infection, we do not always understand why some people become infected and others do not.

Modern physics teaches us that things do not happen to us; things just *are*, and they are waiting for us to give them meaning and life through our perceptions. The fact was that my clock fell off the wall, but the *meaning* of the fall was up to me. What happens is "just the way it is," but such an orientation does not imply surrender. Rather, recognizing and feeling "the way it is" helps us try to become more a conscious part of that "way." We cannot tell the universe what to do, but we can try to get more in step with what it is doing with us. See illness as data of divinity, not predictor of doom, and you have taken the first step to observing illness and crisis in such a way as to create a climate where wellness and healing can show themselves.

Second, tell people in crisis that they do not have to have a "positive attitude" to resolve their problems. Feeling depressed, panicked, helpless, and angry are as important healing feelings as hope, happiness, and laughter. The principle of complementarity teaches us that there is a dualistic aspect that is natural to everything. Being up and down, happy and sad, hopeful and despairing are all important to living through the turmoil of crisis or illness.

When we are sick, we must more than ever before be ourselves and find our "way." We must realize that we are in charge of how we will view the world. We do not have to pretend to be what we are not. As one of the MMs said, "I can't deal with any more meditation and imagery and crystals and vitamins. I can't get a personality transplant and a bone marrow transplant at the same time. I've got to find and be my way. It takes all my time and energy just trying to be me while all of this is going on."

Finally, tell people who are ill or in crisis that there are remarkable laws of life that can help them make miracles. Tell them that they can make their own miracles not by employing imagery, mind-over-matter principles, meditation, cultivating a happy attitude, eating a macrobiotic diet, or taking a guilt trip back to the parthenogenic life event that caused their illness. Tell them that by applying magnificent theories of the cosmos that alter time, space, and energy they can find their own "way with the way it is." Remind them that their chosen perception of their situation is the hypothesis on which their healing will be based. Instead of the miracle blocker of guilt, we need to feel the power of our nonlocal, collective consciousness, supported by the scientific fact that we are much more than "people particles."

Be Sure to Complement Your Self

Niels Bohr's principle of complementarity further asserts that there are always alternative ways of seeing and interpreting events. Just as the left side of the brain provides information (words, places, rational thought, objectivity, and speech) different from that supplied by the right side (symbols, fantasies, feelings, subjectivity, and sensing), so all of the data that we receive are always characterized by alternative views. The principle of complementarity suggests that one view is always incomplete. This means that when we are sick, we are also getting well. We are adjusting, changing, developing, and evolving. If we view defeating physical death as the sole criterion for successful healing, we are doomed to failure. If we view illness from the complementarity principle point of view, we see sickness as only one side of wellness. We do not damn ourselves or our bad luck for being sick. Instead, we realize that we all get sick and suffer, and that our local pain is only one phase of the natural chaos of the cosmos. For every star that is burning out, another is burning brighter, and there can be no health without the developmental adjustments of illness and healing. Even at the most severe times of hurting, we must remember the "other side," the fact that we have the capacity for ultimate joy and spiritual development even through our struggles. The more we feel local pain, the more we must be aware of our potential for cosmic joy.

I never felt more alive than when I was dying. I never felt more joy than when I was crying. I never felt more hope than when things seemed so hopeless. I never felt so connected as when I was alone and feeling the power of the prayers and support of those who love me. The principle of complementarity suggests that happiness and unhappiness always exist together. Even though we are taught that we should strive to achieve happiness and avoid unhappiness, this view ignores the complementarity of each state.

A study by Professor Fausto Massimini at the University of Milan revealed that paraplegics (people unable to move their legs or their arms) viewed the accident that resulted in their paralysis as *both* one of the most negative *and* positive aspects of their lives.[19] They kept sight of the complementary side of their crises, often describing their misery at one time and the fact that they felt reborn, more mature, and closer to God at other times.[20] Like the miracle makers in these studies, so long as I remained open to "the other side of the issue" and refused to accept the old Newtonian "single cause" explanation of life occurrences, the complementary feelings, thoughts, and beliefs about my illness and healing always came to the fore.

"This is really going to hurt," said the nurse as she began the flow of a burning chemical into my vein. "Well, then, it will probably be a tremendous feeling when it doesn't hurt," I said with squinted eyes, tight lips, and shaking body. I tried desperately to focus on the parts of my body that felt good. My wife stroked my back gently and held my hand, and we both focused on the sensations accompanying our embrace. As painful as the chemical was, the pleasure of my wife's touch seemed capable of matching the pain. I never before in my life have known the complementary side of pain so intensely. I never knew the joy of nonpain until I had felt such terrible pain during my treatments. Had I succumbed totally to the local pain, that is all I would have experienced. By looking for the complementary side of pain, the joy of the removal of pain, I was not trapped by my treatments into the role of a suffering victim.

The Certainty of Uncertainty

If Niels Bohr's principle of complementarity disproved the Newtonian notion of singular causation, physicist Werner Heisenberg's uncertainty principle disproved the mechanistic concept of Newtonian determinism. Newton thought that the cosmos could be explained as a carefully balanced set of "things" moving in predictable ways though "space." Heisenberg proved that all of our existence is indeterminate and always just beyond our grasp. The more we know about one thing, the more we can be sure that we do *not* know about something else. According to the uncertainty principle, the lumps of matter and jumps in energy that make up our world are not only complementary sides of a larger picture but as soon as we focus with certainty on a specific lump or particle, we preclude an experience of the "jump" or energy aspect of this lump. We always become uncertain (whether we know it or not) about the complementary aspect of whatever it is we are thinking about or focusing on. If we pay attention only to energy, we ignore particles. According to scientist Erick Jantsch, it is this very inde-terminism and openness of the quantum world that gives our universe its potential for the unexpected, the new, the creative, the miraculous.[21]

The most drastic example of the uncertainty principle in my own illness was what I called the "specialist syndrome." I was examined and treated by specialists from more than fourteen medical areas. Each specialist said essentially the same thing. "I only know my area of expertise." As the old saying goes, my doctors were busy learning more and more about less and less and in my case ended up knowing everything about nothing. They forgot what the un-certainty principle teaches: that in any known situation, there must be another side that is being totally ignored and about which there is no certainty at all.

Even the so-called holistic doctor who treated me was so focused on my "general well-being" that he was unable to be specific enough to diagnose my localized cancer. He was confident in his certainty that "what you need is more vitamins, meditation, and relaxation. You must become more centered." Had he added, "Of course, something very specific and identifiable may be wrong, so we had better focus there, too," I might have been spared eight months of agony.

Whenever you are in a crisis, remember the application of the four new science principles outlined here:

- Remember that *nonlocality*, or "simultaneous action at a dis-tance," is possible, so we are not limited by the here and now. We are everywhere with everyone at the same time. Miracles are possible because we are not limited by time or space.

- Remember that the act of our observation (*observer partici-pantcy*) creates what is observed. The crises in our lives have their impact according to how we choose to see them.

- Remember that there is an infinite duality or *complementarity* to everything in the universe, an up for every down and a step forward to every step backward. Through all of our local pain, there is always cosmic joy waiting for us.

- Remember that the more you or anyone focuses on or "knows" one part of something, the more another side of that something cries out for knowing (*uncertainty*). Making miracles does not require arrogant confidence. What is needed is a humble recognition that in our uncertainty there is always hope.

Beyond the Lonely Brain

Miracles and *meaningful coincidences* are the daily evidence of the four new science principles described above. My "miracle of tears" described earlier in this chapter is only one of many miracles during my "fatal" illnesses. Miracles and coincidences are the clear and indisputable evidence of the fact that we are much more than highly tuned machines with electronic brains who live our few years and then die and decay. I have long known that to be true and have been further convinced of it by my work with the MMs and with hundreds of dying patients. Now, I have been there myself.

Miracles and the meaningful coincidences of our lives are the evidence of our immortality: They prove that we are "soul" and not just "stuff." They attest to the fact that we have a mind as well as a brain. Our physical brains are too local, too simple, too selfish, too immediate, too judgmental to fully know our minds because our brains follow the laws of Newton's mechanical universe. The mind follows the laws of the stars. There is nothing paranormal, New Age, or occult about the fact that our self cannot be localized as one brain in one skull. In fact, our self is shared with all of the souls in the universe. I promise you that someday, at some miraculous moment, you will collect your own data supporting the fact that we are "nonlocal."

"On the first day on the bone marrow transplant floor, we were all alone in our rooms," said one of my fellow transplant patients. "After a few days, we seemed to merge into a unit. It was sudden, and it just happened. We would see each other at X ray or during some treatment or we would receive phone calls intended for one another as if all the calls were coming to all of us. One night, there must have been more than ten calls to the wrong room, even though the callers knew the correct numbers. Once we saw it happening, we worked to be a unit. We thought of each other and listened for each other in the night. We could sense when one of us was in trouble, because we all seemed in trouble. They always use the phrase 'come together' in a sexual way, but we came together by coincidence in every way."

Help Wanted: Inquire Within

At the point of the miracle and the meaningful coincidence *religion and science can merge into one powerful reminder of our divinity.* Our personal experience of our world remains highly spiritual in nature, even though we are drawn through life by our delight in the marvels of scientific technology. We may depend on our personal computer, but in our private moments, we long for a larger, meaningful context for these marvels. We appreciate the convenience brought to us by science, but even as we type, drive, and play with our gadgets, we find ourselves asking "Why?" and "Isn't there more?" There is some instinct within us that pushes us to inquire where we as individuals fit into the collective experience of humankind and the universe. It seems that there is something within us all that senses that we are not limited to one location, one body, and one physical lifetime.

One of my patients asked, "Am I the only one who looks in the mirror in the morning and sometimes thinks 'Hey, that isn't really me. I'm much *more* than that.' Am I the only one who feels sort of out of my self when I see or hear my self? It's as if my soul were taking a look at me and almost laughing at the silly understatement of itself. I seem so insignificant sometimes that my image in the mirror seems like a costume for my soul."

All of us have felt "out of our selves" at one time or another. That sense of infinite self can happen anytime, anyplace—even while we shave or put on makeup. Meaningful coincidences and miracles take place at such times. One woman MM said,

I have what I call my SAC or self-awareness chamber. It's my bathroom. No one is ever in there with me but me. I can think, study my image, look at myself naked. Sometimes, when I really look and think about my body as compared to "me," I have to sit down on my porcelain "meditation chair" in my self-awareness chamber to get back to the everyday world. Maybe I should say I sort of get myself back to being a "part" instead of my whole so I can function in the daily world. If I didn't do that, I think I would sit in there all day and celebrate the magnificence of the irrelevance of my body and the grandeur of my "self."

When I first saw myself naked after my surgeries and chemotherapy, I felt sadness for my body. It had tried so hard for "me," and now it was hurting me and itching me, and it looked beaten, bruised, and bald. My body was taking the brunt of the mechanical approaches to my cure. I saw that my skin was what author and poet Diane Ackerman calls "a feeling bubble" and a "kind of space suit in which we maneuver though an atmosphere of . . . obstacles of all sorts."[22]

As I studied my body and skin, I realized how much *more* than this body I really am and that miracles did not depend on just the state of my body. Miracles take place at the level of the self. Our self is a nonlocal, collective soul, and science proves this fact as strongly as our faith convinces us of it.

The Miracle of Coincidence Clusters

I had just finished lecturing to 4,000 scientists and doctors about the miracles that had accompanied my cure from two cancers. I had been shy about talking so openly about issues that seemed so radical and so unlike the scientist's role that my audience expected of me. As my lecture ended, the room was silent. I thought, "Well, that's it. My career is over and my reputation is ruined. I know I'm telling the truth about these miracles and I know that the scientific principles of nonlocality, observer participantcy, complementarity, and uncertainty on which these miracles are based are valid, but the world just is not ready to hear this material from someone like me."

Then, slowly at first, applause began to spread through the room. Within moments, the entire audience was on its feet not only applauding but cheering and crying. I began to cry and tried to make a graceful exit that would hide my tears. Before I could leave the lecture hall, however, I was surrounded by doctors, nurses, teachers, and other professional people from the audience. Each person wanted to relate their own miracle story. The following doctor's report was typical.

"I don't believe in this stuff, but I want to tell you about something weird that happened to me," he began. (This is the typical introduction to reports about meaningful coincidences and seems to be a strategy designed to distance people from facts that they can never fully deny. However, we are all participant observers, and on some level, we all believe in "weird stuff" when it comes to seeking meaning in our own lives.) He continued,

> Before I give medical treatments to my patients, I always run blood chemistries to be sure that the patient will tolerate the medications I prescribe without complications. However, I have one patient now who refuses to allow me to draw blood each time I give him his medicine. Six times in a row, he said he knew his blood levels. He gave me the numbers and insisted that I write them down. Then he allowed me to draw his blood, and six times in a row he was exactly right on every number. These days, he lets me draw blood every third time just to be sure, but he is always right. And do you want to know what is even stranger? He can tell me a week ahead what his blood levels will be. Now, a lot of my patients can do this same thing. Some of them can even predict to the exact number what their blood chemistry will be. I think it is all just a coincidence, but I thought you would want to know about it.

This physician did not realize that he was changing the way he saw blood chemistry. He had altered his local, mechanical view that there was only one way to determine blood values, and now his world was complying with his viewpoint. He was reluctantly taking part in miracle making, because what he was now willing to see, he could now get.

When I speak on how scientific principles such as observer participantcy can prove the existence of miracles, it seems to legitimize the open examination of the coincidences and ironies in our lives. People seem attracted to these issues, and "coincidence clusters" often form: groups of people experiencing more and more coincidences. I have noticed that whenever I speak about the meaning of coincidences, more and more coincidences seem to occur for me and for those around me. Author Alan Vaughan points out that when one becomes interested in synchronicities or meaningful coincidences, such occurrences seem to multiply![23] He referred to the "synchronicity of synchronicity" and proposed that attention to our nonlocality, the role of our observation, and our capacity for making miracles seems to lower the threshold for such phenomena to occur.

Classifying Your Coincidences

"Dr. Pearsall, Dr. Pearsall!" shouted a woman running toward me in the Chicago airport. "I just saw you on television, and I must tell you about my own coincidence." I had some time before my flight departed for Detroit, so as we walked together, she reported the following story: "I have flown in four crop dusters today. This will be the fifth small plane I've taken today. By remarkable coincidence, I was given seat 7A on the first four flights. I'm going to get my seat assignment now. Please wait to see if it's 7A. I don't know what it means, but it seems really strange and somehow important."

The woman was out of breath, and her eyes searched mine. "I know you probably think I'm weird, but you just have to wait with me to see if I'll get 7A a fifth time. I never *ask* for any given seat. I just got this same seat every time. It must mean something."

This woman's destination, Traverse City, Michigan, was on the gate sign right in front of us, so we stepped over and I waited in the short line with her until she got to the counter. We both laughed as we sensed a nervousness and shared a hope for something neither of us articulated, but both of us knew. We both seemed to sense that this silly coincidence could offer "divine data" that life was more than a meaningless local journey.

The woman assigning seats never looked up. She took my new friend's ticket, typed some codes on her computer, and handed the ticket back. On the jacket, scrawled in green pen, was a check mark. "But what seat do I have?" asked my new friend, shoving her ticket back at the agent.

"It's unassigned seating on this plane," replied the agent. "Just take any seat you like."

My friend looked at her ticket in dismay. "I guess I'll take seat 7A. I hope nobody else takes it first." She seemed disappointed. "I guess four times in a row in 7A was coincidence enough. I'm going to be thinking about what this means during the whole flight."

As she headed toward the boarding ramp, she gave me a quick hug. "Keep telling them about miracles," she said. "They're all over the place if we can just learn to see and read them. I guess they don't always live up to our simple expectations of how they should be, but they're everywhere. Like children, they may not be all you thought they should be, but they usually are all that they can be."

I bent to pick up my luggage and headed for my gate. I looked up at the television screen listing flight departures and scanned down the column until I saw my flight: Detroit—Departing on Time—Gate 7A.

I hope my airport friend reads this. In the next chapter, I will show you that such coincidences can even be classified: This woman's four coincidental same-seat assignments added to my 7A gate assignment would be called a "concurrence of the fifth order." My friend might also be interested to know that I occupied room 7A during my first bone marrow test. I hope she will realize—as I will describe in more detail in the following chapters—that meaningful coincidences are contagious! Synchrony leads to more synchrony because when our consciousness is drawn to our nonlocality and oneness with the universe our energy becomes focused and the way is paved for miracles.

Coincidences are the quantum energy jumps of our lives, manifestations of the fifth energy that holds our universe together. They are quick glimpses through the fog of daily chaos. The first step in making more miracles happen in our lives is to learn to be "miracle literate." We must learn to view coincidences not as random, flukey events but as meaningful indicators of our nonlocality. They teach us that spontaneity is possible (nonlocality); that paying attention to coincidences creates more coincidences, because seeing creates what is seen (observer participantcy); that even as we move through our daily see-and-touch world, there is always the presence of the energy of worlds "on the other side" (complementarity principle); and that as soon as we are certain about our lives, we will be surprised by the synchronicities that draw our attention to the mysterious workings of our spiritual lives (uncertainty principle).

A Chronicle of Coincidences

I suggest that you keep a record of the coincidences in your own life. Write them down as soon as you can after you experience them. Like dreams (and like electrons in the cloud chambers in physics laboratories), the meaningful coincidences of our lives seem to blur and even vanish from our recollection after they happen. Like dreams, meaningful coincidences always seem to come from nowhere and occur with spontaneity and suddenness. Like dreams, meaningful coincidences always have some basis in and grow from our experience, however veiled this basis may be upon first examination.

Coincidences tease us by popping up around us; then, like playful gremlins, they hide from us again. Hawaiians refer to the *menehunes,* or "the invisible little people," who make themselves known briefly and then vanish. Like a cosmic game of hide and seek, the meaningful synchronicities of our lives are perpetual challenges to our willingness to adopt an uncommon consciousness. When you look at your record of your own coincidences, you will in time see the pattern of the four scientific principles outlined in this chapter.

Look first for the overriding scientific principle of our *nonlocality*. Notice the spontaneity of the coincidences in your life and the way in which the limits of time and space seem to be transcended. For example, a friend whom you have not seen for years may call just when you were thinking of that friend, and time and space will have been traversed instantaneously by the connecting of your consciousness with that of your friend.

Examine your coincidences for the impact of your own *observation* on your life. Coincidences happen most often when transitions and crises are in progress, so focus on thoughts of your career, and you may receive a call from someone about a job opportunity or change. View the opportunity as positive to your own development, and the coincidence of a clue to just the right job at the right time might occur.

Study your coincidences for evidence of the *complementarity principle*. Your coincidences will reveal that your life is always a work in progress, and that there is always a side of your living that you have been ignoring. Like the woman in the airport, you may see numbers, themes, or patterns that tell you about something in your past or future that has been neglected. Was this woman ignoring the fact that she was traveling too much, too fast, and too often? Was she traveling through time so quickly that she was catching up with herself and finding herself in the same seat? What metaphor was revealed through her 7A coincidence?

Remember that the more a coincidence seems to mean to you,

there is an opposite and contrasting message hidden somewhere for you to discover. Don't be deceived by its first and obvious meaning. The coincidence of the perfect job interview landing in your lap might draw your attention to the need to spend more time with your family. Your tendency will be to see the coincidences of your life from your present view of your life, but the real value of these coincidences is to jar your attention to the possibility of changing your point of view. If you see a message about your thriving health, for example, look for illness threats and examine your prevention strategies. If you see a message about love, look to the areas of loneliness in your life. The complementarity principle teaches us that the whole picture of life is revealed to us only one side of a life-page at a time, and it takes many two-sided pages to make a complete life story.

Expect the *uncertainty principle* to kick into action as you learn from your coincidences. This means that for every hint you receive in the patterns of your coincidences, you may feel *more* confused. The more you seem to learn, the more you may feel you do not know. Rather than trying to settle things down, use this uncertainty as an invitation to broaden your thinking about life. Perhaps the recurring 7A seat assignment in the businesswoman's coincidence was a mischievousness of the cosmic laws as they awarded this busy woman with a permanent place in flight, hoping to draw to her attention that she was doing too much too fast.

Seeing Better in the Dark

When my oldest son was almost three years old, I remember finding him desperately crawling around the floor in the kitchen. "I lost my truck," he cried, and scurried on. "I thought you were playing with your truck in the front room," I said. "I think you lost it in there." His answer reveals our own failure and fear to look in the right places for the meaning of the chance occurrences in our life. "I know I lost it out there in the dark," he said, looking afraid as he gestured toward the shadowy and more mysterious front room. "I'm looking here because there is more light."

When a coincidence occurs, your quantum world is shaking. An energy wave may be becoming a particle as a thought about a person turns into that person who is making a surprise visit. A particle may be turning into a wave of energy as an unexpected gift results in a flood of long-lost feelings and memories. When you pay attention to the shaking instead of shying away from it, you become a part of and help to create the vibrations of the cosmos.

That is why you are a part of every coincidence in your chronicle. You are both cause and effect. If you look carefully, you will see that your coincidence chronicle will point the way to where the miracles of your life are waiting to be made.

Candles, Clocks, and Beetles

At the beginning of this chapter, I described the coincidence of our clock falling from our wall just before a terrible call arrived from my oncologist. Therapeutic literature is full of such reports of significant moments in persons' lives being accompanied by the occurrence of synchronicities. In fact, it is difficult to find a significant success story taking place in psychotherapy without some coincidence taking place during the therapy.

Years ago, one of my therapy clients was discussing her failure to make peace with her father. They had spent their years together locked in constant argument and struggle for power, and both of them had failed to speak of the love that often smolders under such intense conflict. "I'm so afraid he will die before I ever tell him that I love him," sobbed my patient. At that very moment, both she and I could smell a burned-out candle. Our search revealed no source of the odor. We returned to our therapy and my patient called her father from my office and said, "I'm coming to your house. I want to tell you I love you. It won't be easy, so I'm warning you now of what I might not be able to say to your face." Our session continued for a period of time following this phone call until much relieved, my patient left my office. Hours later, she called me in tears. "My father died while I was with you in my therapy hour. They said he was having chest pains. He's been terribly sick for years. Thank God I took a chance and told him I loved him. He must have been dying when we smelled that burned-out candle. He must have been trying to reach me before he died."

Psychologist Carl Jung suggests that the psychotherapeutic, transformational, deeply emotional, and introspective processes focus our consciousness to help it act as a catalyst for the release of the fifth energy. This energy plays itself out through the synchronicities served up as metaphors for therapeutic progress. My falling clock and the odor of the burned-out candle are examples of this energy-generating process.

To illustrate his point about the power of self-evaluation and struggling for insight to elicit meaningful coincidences, Jung described what psychologists view as the classic example of a psychological synchronicity—or what he called "creative acts . . . acausal parallelism . . . meaningful coincidences."[24] A highly rational and defensive patient of Jung was struggling with the symbolisms and metaphors that are a key part of most psychotherapy. She described a dream in which a golden scarab flew around her shoulders. Jung knew that this type of beetle was valued by the ancient Egyptians as a symbol of renewal and rebirth. As the woman described her dream, a tapping was heard at the window. The tapping continued, so Jung rose to open the window to see what was making the noise. In flew a gold-green beetle. When Jung showed his patient the beetle, her rationalizations and defensiveness to symbolic interpretation were reduced and therapy proceeded at a productive pace. As Jung himself pointed out, "Evidently something quite irrational was needed which was beyond my powers to produce."[25] The coincidence of the golden beetle filled that need.

Scientific writer David Peat notes, "Synchronicities are the jokers in nature's pack of cards for they refuse to play by the rules and offer a hint that, in our quest for certainty about the universe, we may have ignored some vital clues."[26] The burned candles, falling clocks, and golden beetles of our lives are our cosmic clues that anything can happen anytime and anywhere. When we give meaning to these significant surprises, we begin the process of miracle making.

NOTES

1. The description of *synchronicity* as "finding meaning and giving prominence in our lives to the dramatic chance occurrences that take place" is found in Arnold Mindel, "Synchronicity: An Investigation of the Unitary Background Patterning Synchronous Phenomena," *Dissertation Abstracts International* 37:2 (1976). See also C. G. Jung, "Syn-

chronicity: An Acausal Connecting Principle," *Collected Works*, Vol. 8 (Princeton, NJ: Princeton University Press, 1973).

2. For a careful and clear discussion of the statistical explanation of a coincidence such as a hand of all clubs in bridge, see Barry Singer, "To Believe or Not to Believe," in *Science and the Paranormal: Probing the Existence of the Supernatural*, ed. George O. Abell and Barry Singer (New York: Charles Scribner's Sons, 1981), 7–23.

3. Quoted in Allan Combs and Mark Holland, *Synchronicity: Science, Myth, and the Trickster* (New York: Paragon House, 1990), v. This is the best current book that reviews the science, myth, and meaning of meaningful coincidences. It describes many of the same scientific principles outlined in this book as they may be applied to understanding synchronicities.

4. A description of the evolutionary significance of our finding of meaning in our coincidences is found in B. F. Skinner, "The Force of Coincidence," *The Humanist* 37, no. 3 (1977): 10–12.

5. Richard M. Bucke, *Cosmic Consciousness* (New York: Dutton, 1969), 10.

6. Quoted in Clifford A. Pickover, *Computers, Pattern, Chaos, and Beauty: Graphics from an Unseen World* (New York: St Martin's Press, 1990), 141.

7. Larry Dossey, *Recovering the Soul: A Scientific and Spiritual Search* (New York: Bantam Books, 1989), 17–19.

8. *Ibid.*, 18.

9. For a thorough discussion of the danger to our survival posed by the refusal of establishment medicine and the vested interest of big drug companies to consider alternative approaches to treating serious illness (for example, the rejection of vitamin C therapy by the National Cancer Institute), see John M. Fink, *Third Opinion* (New York: Avery Publishing Group, 1988).

10. Quoted in William Safire and Leonard Safire, *Words of Wisdom* (New York: Simon & Schuster, 1989), 39.

11. Dossey, *Recovering the Soul*, 19.

12. Harold J. Morowitz, *Cosmic Joy and Local Pain. Musings of a Mystic Scientist* (New York: Charles Scribner's Sons, 1987), 300.

13. *Ibid.*, 303.

14. For a discussion of the relationship between the theories of quantum mechanics and their impact on our daily life and beliefs, see Ken Wilbur, ed., *Quantum Questions: Mystical Writings of the World's Great Physicists* (Boston: New Science Library, 1984).

15. Dana Zohar, *The Quantum Self: Human Nature and Consciousness Defined by the New Physics* (New York: William Morrow, 1990), 25.

16. Ms. Hay's book has been a popular reference for people with serious illnesses. I feel that the book can engender guilt and self-blame in suffering patients, but it is a work that challenges the simple mind/body separation of traditional medicine. See Louise L. Hay, *You Can Heal Yourself* (Santa Monica, CA: Louise Hay, 1984).

17. John White, *The Meeting of Science and the Spirit* (New York: Paragon Books, 1990), 99.

18. Quoted in Jay W. Haywood, *Perceiving Ordinary Magic* (Boulder, CO: Shambhala, 1984), 174.

19. This work was translated by Mihaly Csikszentmihalyi, *Flow: The Psychology of Optimal Experience* (New York: HarperCollins, 1990), 193.

20. *Ibid.*, 195. Csikszentmihalyi describes studies of blind persons and others with life-altering crises who report the complementary side of their challenge. In our pursuit of happiness, we often lose sight of the fact that it is right there beside our unhappiness.

21. Erick Jantsch, *The Self-Organizing Universe* (New York: Pergamon, 1980).

22. Diane Ackerman, *A Natural History of the Senses* (New York: Random House, 1990), 67.

23. A. Vaughan, *Incredible Coincidence* (Philadelphia: Lippincott, 1979).

24. C. G. Jung and W. Pauli, *The Interpretation and Nature of the Psyche*, trans. R. F. C. Hull and P. Silz (New York: Pantheon, 1955).

25. C. Jung, "Synchronicity: An Acausal Connecting Principle," *Collected Works*, vol. 8 (Princeton, NJ: Princeton University Press, 1973), 23.

26. David Peat, *Synchronicity: The Bridge Between Matter and Mind* (New York: Bantam Books, 1988), 7.

3
THE NATURE AND NURTURING OF MIRACLES

Learning to Read Miracle Maps

God never wrought miracles to convince atheism, because His ordinary works convince it.
—FRANCIS BACON

Moving Between Heaven and Earth

When I was dying, I remembered how I used to feel when I hid in a
closet as a little boy. I would become terrorized by the complete
silence and darkness as I huddled within the clothing. I felt like I
was being swallowed up by the heavy dark coats and pants that I
could not see. It was the first time in my life that I was totally
unable to see and that I encountered the complete silence caused
by the soundproofing of layers of cloth. Even though everything
was black, it seemed that I could look down and see myself
crouched in that closet. When my death seemed certain, I felt like I
was back in that closet again.

I remember my father opening the closet door and hugging me. I
remember the rush of fresh air and, like exiting a tunnel, a burst of
overwhelming light as both my father and I won our game of hide

and seek. I remember that my father seemed to know why I was crying and why I wouldn't leave his side the rest of the day. When my father died suddenly years later, I remember praying that he never felt the fear and loneliness of that dark closet. When I faced my own death now as an adult, the memory of that closet was strong, yet I also felt an overwhelming presence that seemed ready to welcome me. I saw the dark tunnel with the light at the end that so many people who have faced death describe. I saw and heard deceased relatives calling to me and comforting me, and I hoped my father had felt that same solace.

Psychiatrist Raymond Moody published the earliest studies of near-death experiences (NDEs).[1] He includes several actual stories recounted by persons who have survived dying, and each story shows the same elements I experienced.

NDEs are not uncommon. Pollster George Gallup, Jr., reports that nearly 5 percent of the adult population in North America has had a near-death experience.[2] Like my experience, such incidences are not dreamlike. The person tends to feel *more* alert, awake, and insightful than ever before. The dark tunnel effect and a contrasting yellow-orange light are typically experienced; deceased friends and relatives are seen and sometimes heard; there is the pervasive feeling of levitating, and a choice often has to be made as to whether or not to return to terrestrial life. I experienced every one of these phenomena each time I faced my own death, and every one of my seventeen miracle-making patients reported these same experiences as well.

A few months after my NDE, I was sorting through my slides to prepare a lecture when "by coincidence" I came across a reproduction of the painting by Hieronymus Bosch called *The Ascent of the Blessed*. The painting depicts souls ascending to heaven through a long tunnel with a light at the end. I recognized the painting immediately as reflective of my own experiences. I recognized the nonlocality and cosmic quality of the work as the same ambience of my own NDE. In keeping with the observer participantcy principle, the painting seemed to suggest that the souls themselves were creating their own experience through their own visions. I saw in the painting the "other sidedness" or complementarity of living and dying. I saw the delightful wonder and uncertainty in the faces in that work of art, and I realized that all four of the principles of

science described earlier in this book were depicted in this painting of the transition of dying that I had "just happened" to notice.

Delusion or Divinity?

Like many scientists, writer Arthur Koestler felt that near-death
experiences are forms of delusional death throes that serve the
purpose of saving us from facing the infinite of emptiness that
inevitably follows our brief local existence. He wrote of people like
me who had NDEs: "Their minds went haywire and saturated the
atmosphere with ghosts of the dead and other invisible presences
who at best were inscrutable."[3]

Despite numerous published reports describing NDEs in pres-
tigious medical journals,[4] most scientists dismiss the significance
of NDEs as similar to drug-induced hallucination. They feel that
NDEs are due to "perceptual release," or the brain's surrender to its
memories and fantasies as a result of decreased external stimulation, accompanied by increased awareness caused by fear, drugs,
and other physiological aspects of impending death.[5]

I have no doubt that, on one level of reality, NDEs are indeed
hallucinations, but this does not mean that the hallucinations
themselves have no meaning! Just as the fact that coincidences can
be predicted and explained by statistical tables does not mean that
they cannot have significance on several levels beyond statistical
reality, so near-death experiences (hallucinatory or not) are our
business as much as science's business.

The patterns and commonalities of NDEs and the fact that very
young children never exposed to prior reports of the NDE also
report much the same characteristics in their own NDEs indicates
that there are many ways of understanding the nature of our
confrontation with our mortality. Many researchers have come to
view such occurrences as being valid, significant, and explainable
by the laws of new science. For example, the nonlocality of our
consciousness—the fact that our mind is not just in our brain and
that we are much more than our molecular pattern—is supported
by neurosurgeon Wilder Penfield. Penfield failed throughout his
career to explain human consciousness merely in terms of the
brain's electrochemical processes. He came to think that the mind
exists independently of the physical brain.[6]

Scientists are more comfortable calling the spiritual and nonlocal aspects of our NDEs "autoscopic visions." By this they mean that subjects (like the blind patient I described in the previous chapter) report floating up and out of their physical form to see details of their surroundings. Cardiologist Michael Sabom has studied several independently confirmed autoscopic experiences. He concludes, "I do believe, however, that the observations . . . concerning the autoscopic NDE indicate that this experience cannot be casually dismissed as some mental fabrication, and that serious scientific consideration must be given to alternative, perhaps less traditional explanations."[7]

The scientific evidence supporting our nonlocality also supports the idea that NDEs shouldn't be dismissed as the hopeless last mental gasps of a short-circuiting brain. Instead, NDEs might well be evidence that there is no need for a last gasp at all unless it is a gasp of awe at our capacity to cast our mind into the realm of our immortality. NDEs are both neurophysiological reflexes *and* coincidences—miracles that prove our cosmic connection.

Which Miracle to Choose?

After a nearly fatal automobile accident, anthropologist Patrick Gallagher was comatose for weeks. His story of his own NDE contains the often-reported sense of levitation, the light and the tunnel, the welcoming friends and relatives, the sense of unity with the universe and of being all-knowing. He also describes the key element of NDE that has *not* been focused on, but it is a key to the making of our own miracles.

Each time that I confronted my own death, *I was also confronted with a choice*. I felt such peace, profound knowledge, and merging with lost loved ones that I struggled with the decision to return to my earthly life. I was experiencing what my MMs had reported: that they had to choose their miracle. They had to resolve their uncertainty between two complementary miracles or points of view: to experience life "here" and locally or to merge with an infinite everywhere with everyone.

Gallagher describes his own choice. He writes, "I knew it was quite possible to return to my terrestrial life, and I missed . . . my children, my wife, and many others. I did decide to return, though

I knew also that the price of the ticket would be gargantuan; accepting the biological, physiological, and physical needs and handicaps of my body, as well as the loss of all but a splinter of my luminous knowledge."[8] In a sense, we all have NDEs every day. We all make choices as to how our life should be. We all select our miracles by choosing a miraculous point of view about the major transitions in our life. We all choose to heed or ignore the daily coincidences that hint at the larger meaning of these transitions.

There are *minor* coincidences or miracles such as the chance assignment of a seat on an airplane described in chapter 2. There are *meaningful* coincidences that relate to our choice of a place to live and whom to love. And there are the *magnificent* miracles and coincidences such as my own coming back from physical death. If we pay attention to our miracles, we see that some choice is always required. In acknowledgment of our "observer" power, we may make a simple choice between airplane seats in an attempt to maintain some pattern amid apparent disorder. In acknowledgment of the uncertainty of life, we might decide to try for a job based on a quick glance at a want ad that seems to demand our attention just when we were certain that we would never discover such a lead. Or perhaps we must choose between living locally or returning spiritually to move within the cosmos. All miracles and coincidences are calls for a choice between a life of uncommon consciousness and the more common consciousness of a simple, mechanical, cause-and-effect world view.

Big Bangs, Little Booms, and God's Laws

In his essay "Of Miracles," philosopher Baruch Spinoza writes that if miracles were exceptions to cosmic law, then God's existence would be disproved.[9] But miracles do not break God's laws. They are evidence of the action of His laws. To see coincidences as miracles—as moments of insight into the workings of cosmic laws—is to see daily evidence of the work of God.

The transitions of birth, life, and death are the miraculous "big bangs" of the cosmic laws; they are curtain calls in the infinite drama of the coming and going of our collective spirit to what scientist and philosopher Guy Murchie calls "soul school."[10] All that is "permanent" in the cosmos are the patterns, changes, energy fields, forms, forces, and rules of transcendence and transformation of the universe, not the "stuff" that we see in the mirror in our "self-awareness chamber." Scientists Frank Wilczek and Betsy Devine write, "Matter itself is capable of drastic transformations at all levels, down to and including the most basic. What is conserved, in modern physics, is not any particular substance or material but only much more abstract entities such as energy, momentum, and electric charge."[11] The miracle of who we are, then, is not an unusual miracle. It is natural that changes occur in our life or that we feel the rhythm of being more or less aware of our connection with God. Coincidences and miracles are only glimpses of how closely connected with God we really are.

What is most fascinating is that miracles and coincidences do not just happen to us. We can *make* them happen by being "miracle literate" and using our uncommon consciousness. From the simple redundancy of the 7A seat assignment to the profound near-death experience, we become miracle makers when we choose to seek the meaning of these mysteries of life. As one of my MMs pointed out, "Life deals the hand, but we play it. It's remarkable how different the whole game can be when we realize that you can play a bad deal into a pretty good game." You will be dealt your own coincidences; what you make of them is up to you.

The "little booms" of our life are at least as revealing as the big bangs. What is remarkable is God's willingness to provide us with regular clues to our divinity in our everyday life that are as much evidence of our nonlocality as near-death experience, near-birth experience, and other dramatic changes that take place during the "quantum vibrations" or the transition times of our life when the fifth energy is rearranging itself. Miraclulous coincidences are the aftershocks of our traveling between the realms of reality.

Rainbows at Night

As I travel at night on Maui, I have seen rainbows. Lunar rainbows occur as a result of moisture in the clouds migrating across the Pacific to pause over the mountains of Maui when the moon is near full. These rainbows are silver, with the slightest hint of the spectrum of colors of the solar rainbows. Ancient Hawaiians say that these cosmic silver bands are the demi-god Maui's nighttime reminder that he is still in control of the island.

I wish I had known of these nighttime rainbows when, years ago, I sat with my friend Mike, a doctor on staff at the University of Indiana Medical School. We sat on the steps of the student union building on the campus of Indiana University. It was a warm, muggy evening so common on the southern Indiana campus. Hundreds of poplar trees were silhouetted against a pearl gray sky lit by a full moon. The sweet smell of a huge lilac bush perfumed the air around us. As often happens when we become intoxicated by the majesty, power, and beauty of the natural world, we begin to reflect about our place and purpose in the cosmos.

"I would give anything for one sign. Just one sign that there is really something more," said Mike as he looked at the moon. "Wouldn't it be miraculous if just one clear sign, just one word from God to our ears, could tell the world that He's there—or at least that something is there beyond just *here*. Why does it all have to be blind faith? Why can't we have partially sighted faith?"

I remember hoping that we would see a shooting star at just that moment, but, of course, you often cannot seem to find a miracle just when you need one. If you wait for a miracle, it will never happen. We must learn to make them happen.

"You agree, don't you, Mike, that you are a part of nature, of the world and the universe?" I asked.

"Of course," he responded, still searching the sky. "That's that nonlocal stuff you are always lecturing about. But I'm talking about a real sign, not something philosophical or symbolic."

"Then why don't you get busy sending some signs of your own? You're part of the system, so why don't you start watching for the smallest signs of the miraculous and let everyone know about them? You said you were hoping for just one small sign. Start looking, and I promise you will see many more than one, and sometimes they won't seem so small, either."

Mike knew of my work in the field of miracles and coincidences. Sometimes he jokingly referred to it as "miracology." Tonight, however, he merely looked at me in disbelief and disappointment.

"Paul, I'm talking about a *real* miracle. I need some evidence of our immortality and connection with the cosmos, as you call it. Just one little sign, that's all." He looked down at the steps as if in despair of his search. Suddenly, the bright night sky darkened for an instant, and our moon shadows disappeared. Mike looked up quickly. "It's just a cloud passing in front of the moon," he said looking back down.

"I guess that's not a big enough sign for you," I said.

"You mean that the chance occurrence of a cloud blocking out the moon at just the time we are talking about meaning in the universe is a sign?" he laughed. "In that case, I see thousands of signs a year and maybe dozens every day, and many of them are more impressive than a passing cloud," he continued.

"I rest my case," I said, and we both laughed. "You seem to think that if you see it, then you'll believe it." I continued, "I suggest that if you believe it, you'll probably be better able to see it."

Henry David Thoreau wrote, "The mind can be profaned by the habit of attending to trivial things." We have become used to speed, noise, and the minute-by-minute fireworks of our hectic daily lives. The grandeur of a lunar rainbow and swirling night clouds hiding the moon from us are the lofty parts of our living.

Making miracles is a matter of developing a vigilance for the miracles all around us. If we are open to the miracles right under our very noses, and if we become miracle observers and un-ashamed practioners of miracology, we are, in Thoreau's words, "associating reverently with our loftiest thought." And we are much more likely to participate in the making of our own miracles.

The Baseball Umpire and the Miracle

The umpire was getting tired. The score was fourteen to one, there were two outs, and the losing team was batting in the bottom of the ninth inning. The batter was going through his typical super-stitious dance of hitting his spikes with his bat, spitting on his hands, and caressing his crotch. By the time he stepped into the batter's box, the umpire was about to collapse of fatigue and impatience.

The first pitch sailed past the batter at head level, and the catcher jumped to catch the ball. "Strike one!" yelled the umpire.

"That's not a strike!" screamed the batter. "Who the hell do you think you are, calling that a strike?"

As the laughing catcher threw the ball back to the pitcher, the umpire said, "Out here on the field, I think I'm God. I know I'm the umpire. Nothin' ain't nothin' until I call it. After I call it a strike, it's a strike. Case closed. Batter up!" The umpire's point of view is an example of the impact of observation on living. In effect, we are all calling our own game.

As the umpire says, "Nothin ain't nothin until we call it." There is much more to the game of living than miraculous grand slam home runs in the bottom of the ninth inning. If we wait for only such events, we will miss the joy of the whole game. I suggest that you are the umpire, and how the game is played is your own call.

Why Miracles Are Not Miraculous

Miracles have always constituted the show biz side of religion and have been the target of the science's mockery. I argue for a new balance in the science verses religion debate about miracles. As Albert Einstein wrote, "Religion without science is blind. Science without religion is lame."

Unfortunately, the word *miracle* has gotten a lot of bad press. It has come to mean that God intervenes directly in the operation of his world and breaks his own rules by causing something grand to happen that "can't happen." I suggest that miraculous coincidences are explainable by the laws of new physics. Miracles are not evidence of God breaking his own rules; they are clues about how miraculous God's laws really are and how much a part of these laws we humans are.

We do not have to look for the shock of impossible happenings to find our miracles. Award-winning physicist Niels Bohr, author of the principle of complementarity described in chapter 2, writes, "Anyone who is not shocked by quantum theory has not understood it." What is shocking is that we are offered scientific proof of God's laws. For my money, that is miracle enough. I have lived dozens of miracles, and so have you. There is nothing strange about the fact that we are as much spirit as stuff, as much mind as matter. Science has offered us the proof that we are everything.

UFOnauts and the Flying Saint

A favorite miracle often discussed is that of levitation. I experienced the sensation of hovering over my own deathbed, and all of my MMs report this same feeling at various times during their near-death miracles. Flying saucers are one example of the technicalization and modernization of levitation. Many people have reported seeing unidentified flying objects. Some even report seeing UFOnauts, or the pilots of these machines. Contrary to popular belief, the people giving accounts of UFO sightings are not typically mentally or intellectually impaired. Several scientists and world leaders willing to risk talking of such things publicly have shared their own stories of encounters with UFOs. Former President Jimmy Carter insists that he sighted a UFO, but stopped talking about his experience once he was in office. Several government agencies have made inconclusive studies of the existence of UFOs.[12] All efforts have failed to discourage the public's conviction that levitating machines from outer space visit us from time to time.

The Chinese write that Taoist sages and alchemists were able to rise up into the air. In India, the magical flight of the yogi siddhis is reported. The Buddhists report that flight is a natural ability of the fully enlightened (the arhat).[13] The ability to levitate is attributed to shamans in tribal societies.

Officer Ray Kelly of the Australian Parks and Wildlife Service is an initiate of the Bhungutti, or one of the aboriginal tribal cultures. The most developed of this group, the so-called fourth-stage initiates, are said to have learned to fly. Researcher, musician, artist, and author Richard Heinberg reports that Kelly's uncle saw a fourth-stage tribal member "fly from one mountain to another."[14]

Author and researcher Mircea Eliade reports that some Christian saints were also reported to have levitated.[15] The flying holy brother of the seventeenth century, St. Joseph of Cupertino, was said by several people to have been seen to be flying regularly. A witness recounts: "He rose into space, and, from the middle of the church, flew like a bird onto the high altar, where he embraced the tabernacle. . . . Sometimes, too, he was seen to fly to the altar of St. Francis and of the Virgin of Grotello."[16] Physicist Paul Davies reports that St. Joseph's holy brothers were so embarrassed by his tendency to float in the air at worship that they locked him up in his cell to prevent his aerobatics from disrupting mass.[17]

These and hundreds of other accounts are fascinating stories, and nothing about these stories violates the basic laws of new physics, which confirm that time and space are relative and can be transcended. Almost everyone who has had a NDE has experienced a sense of flying as I did. Whether anyone actually "flew" in the local and mechanical sense of flight is not important. Have you ever felt "light-headed," "flighty," or as if you were floating at some intense time in your own life? There is something within us that is made to fly. The real question scientists should be asking is not just "Are there UFOs?" or "How could levitation be possible?" They should be busy studying which miraculous laws of the cosmos might have been at work during these unusual times and exploring why such events seem so common to many of us. The argument should not be about whether people fly. Rather, study should be made of what it is about us that wants so strongly for our spirits to soar.

The Misguided Miracle

I have referred to three types of miraculous coincidence: minor, meaningful, and magnificent miracles. Minor miracles can often become "misguided" miracles, or what I call abused miracles. Scientists and religious leaders alike often exploit such occurrences to prove their respective points of view. If we are busy using sophisticated machinery to define a vague image of Christ imprinted on a piece of cloth, or praying fervently to see a sacred statue cry, we may miss the amazement on the face of a child and his parents when, during a Christmas Eve reading of "A Visit from St. Nicholas," everyone seems to hear the jingling of sleigh bells on the roof and the sudden but gentle quivering and tinkling of the glass ornaments on the Christmas tree.

Minor miracles become misguided miracles when they are "used" rather than celebrated, debated rather than shared, and often lead to the reaction of "wow" rather than "aha." Misguided miracles are more entertaining than enlightening and divisive rather than unifying. The meaningful miracle, on the other hand, is powerful in its simplicity and commonality.

The Meaningful Miracle

A meaningful miracle takes place when we recognize events that prove our nonlocality. Meaningful miracles are common, simple, and sometimes seem of no apparent relevance at the moment we experience them. Like flashes of lightning unaccompanied by the typical delayed clap of thunder, meaningful miracles are often incomplete and gain significance only in retrospect. Make no mistake: The golden beetle, falling clock, and burned-out candles are just as significant as the flying saint.

If miracles are "unmiraculous," common, and right under our noses, why do so many people refuse to acknowledge their relevance? I believe this is due to our *chosen way of observing* our daily living. I believe we have fallen into Thoreau's "profanity of the trivial" or what philosopher William Irwin Thompson calls a collective hypnosis or cultural trance that prevents us from seeing the basis of our divinity.[18]

The Magnificent Miracle

When we *choose to give* a meaningful miracle a place of influence in our consciousnesses, we elevate it to a "magnificent miracle." God gives us the "stuff" in the form of a chance happening, and we use our own powers to make it come alive and take on meaning in our lives. Now that I have survived several "deaths," I have learned to make a magnificent miracle or two every day of my life. Every chance occurrence, from a lunar rainbow to a hidden moon, offers me a chance to glimpse the universal laws of our life. With such vision, I can see forever and everywhere, and like all of the MMs, I feel much more one with God. I am able to celebrate life as the opportunity to make our meaning out of life's chaos.

As I reported earlier, I am writing this book in my home in Maui. I first became ill here, but I never knew at the time just how sick I would be. I would barely be able to walk through my home without falling to the floor in pain. In keeping with the principle of complementarity, my home in Maui has been my hurting place and my healing place. Now, as I type these words, I can look over my shoulder at Haleakala volcano. As I am typing, I feel a minor earthquake. Such quakes are quite common on the Hawaiian Islands due to the tectonics or shifting of the earth just beneath the ocean waters.

The quake knocked down a picture from my wall near my writing table. It is a picture of my wife and sons. I remember that I have been writing for hours and it is time to be with those whom I love. What a miracle it is to still be with them and to be reminded to love them in such an "earthly" fashion.

The Sistine Chapel Syndrome

My wife and I recently were attending a meeting in Rome, Italy. I was speaking to a large group of insurance salespeople and their spouses. After I completed my lecture about the meaning of miracles, we headed off for a tour of Vatican City.

Michelangelo's work in the Sistine Chapel had just been renovated, and we waited for hours in line for a glimpse of this remarkable feat. When we drew close enough to get a glimpse of the most famous ceiling in the world, I was embarrassed to think, "Gee, that doesn't look so great. Just a bunch of cluttered paintings placed on the ceiling instead of the wall." As the line moved along, people chattered and joked about a paint-by-number replica of Michelangelo's work for their own ceilings.

When we drew closer, however, we were overwhelmed. The paintings seemed to engulf us. Everyone became quiet. Necks ached with the effort to keep looking up. I had not had the right perspective at first, but now I could see and feel the work easily and profoundly. I had been reacting to my own idea about the art, but now that I saw the *artist's reality,* I could not avoid its impact. I felt a part of the paintings. I was a participating observer in the historical tracings of a miracle wrought by an artist who himself had been able to see and represent for us the nature of magnificent miracles.

I noticed a fly crawling across the paintings. I thought, "What a shame. That fly is right up there where I would love to be. He's right on top of it and closer than any of us, but he just can't see it." Then I remembered reading the work of philosopher William Irwin Thompson. When I returned home, I looked up his work and found the following quote:

We are like flies crawling across the ceiling of the Sistine Chapel. We cannot see what angels and gods lie underneath the threshold of our perceptions. We do not live in reality: we live in our paradigms, our habituated perceptions, our illusions, the illusions we share through culture we call reality, but the true . . . reality of our condition is invisible to us.[19]

To avoid these states of "habituated perceptions," we must not keep ourselves too "close" to—or too immersed in—our daily "doing" to remember how to "be" a part of our living. The minor and often misguided miracles that receive press and public attention provide only grounds for debate or entertainment. We must learn to look for meaningful miracles and make them miraculous by fitting them into the choices we make about our living.

The First Collector of Coincidences

Albert Einstein studied work on coincidences completed in 1916 by the Austrian biologist Paul Kammerer. Einstein's assessment of Kammerer's work was that it is "original and by no means absurd." Scientist Arthur Koestler concluded that the work revealed insight into the "integrative tendency of the universe."[20] The great scientific minds of Einstein and Koestler grasped the significance of sudden serendipity as a clue to the organization of our world, yet Kammerer's work has gone essentially ignored for decades.

Kammerer's main point was that coincidences are not random. Coincidences, he felt, were serial and thus related over time and reflective of the relativity theory of the equivalence of time, space, and matter. His statistical analysis of hundreds of coincidences revealed that "There is a basic interconnectedness between things within the deeper patterns of universal laws."[21] We are fascinated by the coincidences of our lives, but we continue to resist their significance as the "signs" that my friend Mike so longed for. A cloud blocking out the moon at just the time when someone is asking for a sign of something miraculous is a miracle if, as one of the MMs said, "we have a lofty literacy."

A Coincidence Classification System

Kammerer devised a system for classifying coincidences.[22] His "coincidence classification system" may help you classify your own coincidences. Take, for example, the story in chapter 2 of the woman in the Chicago airport who was assigned four consecutive 7A seats. Kammerer would have called this a concurrence of the *fourth order* because four related coincidences took place in a series. Review your own coincidences and count the related events. If they are simple consecutive events, Kammerer would have classified them by referring to their "order."

On the other hand, if your synchronous events are not consecutive but "parallel," such as when you think about a friend and that friend calls just at that time, Kammerer referred to such an event as a concurrence of the *first power*. If your friend tells you that she called because she had been dreaming about you the night before, this becomes a concurrence of the *second power*, or two parallel synchronous and meaningful events.

I hope you will try this coincidence classification system in your own life. I suggest that the higher the order or power of your coincidence, the more the universe is trying to draw your attention to some aspect of your living, loving, and believing. In response, consider making some miracles in your own life by applying the lessons of the four basic scientific principles described in chapter 2. In your daily interactions with others, bear in mind your non-locality and connection with everyone and everything. Be aware of the power of your observations of your life. Be alert for alternative and complementary explanations and goals in daily living. Most of all, consider the possibility that you are behaving in too certain a fashion to stay healthy in an uncertain world.

Scientific Fanaticism and Resistance to Miracles

Although nonlocality is a fact that any well-read scientist knows and every religious person senses, to apply such a concept to daily life requires a quantum leap of consciousness that many scientists and religious people seem afraid to take.

One of the MM patients who survived several serious threats to her life was a Sunday school teacher. She was very religious, and when it came to seeing that science and religion could combine to help us make miracles, she said, "What's hard about making miracles is that you have to leap before you look. You have to be willing to think cosmically, quantumly, personally, and spiritually all at one time, and if you try to figure it all out first, you never take the chance to try making miracles. You have to go with the way it is, and the way it is is amazing."

Like the old story of the blind man touching the elephant, the minister and the scientist describe only the part of the elephant on which they have a firm hold. The whole elephant is missed. Meaningful coincidences occur when the whole elephant flashes into our consciousness all at once and we are able to let go of our grip on one small part of the whole.

A classic in the statistical and psychological study of meaningful coincidences is a book by Hans Eysenck and Carl Sargent titled *Explaining the Unexplained*. Carl Sargent reports that one of his colleagues at the University of London called him aside after a thorough presentation of the extensive evidence supporting the existence of meaningful miracles. The colleague said, "The results you presented would convince me of anything else, but this: I just cannot believe it and I don't know why."[23]

This colleague has a firm hold of the elephant's tail, and thinks it's a snake. We simply cannot be so firmly fixed in a local world view and still be able to understand the nature of miracles. Whether we decide to act like the flies on the Sistine Chapel ceiling or learn to soar with the wonderful freedom of our nonlocality is a key choice in whether we make miracles in our lives.

Two years ago, I was visiting England on a book tour. While waiting for my appearance on BBC-TV, I was talking with the producer of the show, which focused on what they called "frontiers in science." I was to discuss my then current book, but the producer had heard of my work in "miracology." She told me that one of their guests more than twenty years ago was the British poet laureate J. B. Priestly. He announced on television that he was conducting a study into coincidences and unusual experiences with time. He invited viewers to send him their own examples of coincidences, and he received thousands of responses. He then had them examined in detail by a panel of scientifically trained and highly skeptical investigators whose primary function was to debunk false scientific reports and attempt to eliminate fraud and carelessness in scientific research. Priestly reported that the panel left him with dozens of reports of meaningful coincidences that it had accepted, somewhat reluctantly, as being scientifically valid.[24]

Physicist Stephen Hawking suggests, "If we were ever to discover a complete theory of cosmology, we might come to know the mind of God."[25] If we can come to grips with our nonlocality as revealed by the miracles of meaningful coincidence, we may learn, as philosopher Spinoza suggests, that we are all "thoughts in the mind of God."[26]

Two Books on "Banging"

More than a quarter of a century ago, William Masters and Virginia Johnson wrote a book titled *Human Sexual Response*.[27] About three years ago, Stephen Hawking wrote the book *A Brief History of Time*. One of my medical students said, somewhat indelicately, "Both of these best-selling books are about banging. Masters and Johnson wrote about local banging and Hawking wrote about cosmic banging, but they are both about the big bang theory of life." By coincidence, my reading of both of these ground-breaking books led me to writing my own books that described practical applications of research findings in sexuality and (now) of physics.

Between Master and Johnson's work and Hawking's book, we have gone from searching for a science of sex to guide us toward fulfillment to a quest for a more cosmic meaning to our short stay on earth. I do not believe that we will find the way to a happy sex life by looking through the lens in the end of a plastic penis vibrating in a vagina. The secret of sexual union is found not within our genitals but within our "selves" and in the interaction between those "selves." Nor do I believe that the meaning of life can be found in theories of the big bang, in images sent back from the Hubble telescope (named after the theorist who suggested the big bang theory), or in scientists' or theologians' debates about the validity of miracles. The answers we seek are revealed to us in the meaningful coincidences of our own everyday experiences which we, if we so choose, may elevate to magnificent miracles.

The Law of Literary Luck

As part of my research for this book, I needed the specific reference for the publisher of Stephen Hawking's book. I could not find it. Someone had borrowed my copy of the book, so I sat back and decided to rest and see if I could remember the publisher on my own. I switched on my tape recorder to listen to what I thought was my favorite Mozart tape. Instead, I heard the voice of Emmy award–winning radio host Michael Jackson presenting the audiocassette version of Hawking's book. Within seconds, he announced the data I needed.

Many authors and researchers have spent hours searching desperately for just the right piece of information, only to have a book fall open to just the page they needed for their information. Well-known author Dame Rebecca West reports that she had spent hours looking for the record of an incident in the Nuremberg trials. She writes,

> I looked up the trials in the library and was horrified to find they are published in a form almost useless to the researcher. They are abstracts, and are catalogued under arbitrary headings. After hours of search I went along the line of shelves to an assistant librarian and said: "I can't find it, there's no clue, it may be in any of these volumes. There are shelves of them." I put my hand on one volume and took it out and carelessly looked at it, and it was not only the right volume, but I had opened it at the right page.[28]

Among ourselves, we refer to the coincidental finding of just the right bit of information as "literary luck."

The rush of wonder and excitement engendered by such coincidences may explain why we will spend hours in libraries for just one big bang of discovery. One author told me, "It's like an orgasm. I get so high when I find something like that that I run home and work for hours." I felt much the same after my chance discovery of the book I mentioned in chapter 2 by Harold Morowitz titled *Cosmic Joy and Local Pain* at just the time when I was experiencing both.

Major breakthroughs in medicine and science are often sparked by meaningful coincidences like the one experienced by Rebecca West. The trick is to *be open enough in your observations* to heed the clue that's being sent your way. Penicillin was discovered by the "accident" of mold being left to grow in an unwashed petri dish in the laboratory. Scientist Jeremy Hayward reports that his choice of a career change from physics to experimental biology happened "coincidentally." He writes,

> I spent several weeks thinking over whether to make a rather big leap from theoretical physics to experimental biology. Walking along

the street, *still uncertain*, I came across a traffic jam and there right in front of me was the bus leading directly to the biology laboratory. I climbed on the bus and reported to the director of the laboratory that I would like to go and work there. That is how *the decision* was made that led to a *tremendous expansion of possibilities* in my life.[29] (italics mine).

Hayward's willingness to accept his uncertainty and his choice to follow the lead of coincidence led to a big bang of discovery and opened up a rich new vein of life.

Monstrous Meaningful Moments

Look back on your life and write down the most significant choices you made. Most of us remember "monstrous moments" when one choice changed our whole future. If you sit quietly and reflect, or if you talk with friends and have them share their own monstrous moments, you will probably discover that a meaningful miracle and coincidence were as significant in your choice as were logical thought and careful reflection. You will learn that you may have made your own miracle by allowing a meaningful coincidence to affect, determine, or explain a major life decision or transition.

I have used this monstrous meaningful moment exercise with many of my patients during my twenty-five years of clinical work. I use it to point out that there is more to living our lives than logical, rational struggles to make decisions. If we pay attention to the natural laws revealed in meaningful miracles, we can give new meaning to the phrase "going with the flow."[30]

A good scientific definition of the meaningful coincidences of our life is provided by Jeremy Hayward: "A meaningful coincidence consists of two simultaneous events that appear to be interconnected, though not by the separate causes that gave rise to them individually."[31] You have seen in this chapter that it is the miracle maker who makes the cosmic connection that gives meaning to our synchronicities. But why is it that some people seem to be better "cosmic connectors" and more skilled readers of miracles than others? Why do some people seem to do so well at making miracles? Why can some people seem to make a miracle for themselves or others just when a miracle is needed the most? I address these issues in the following chapter on the merging of the miracle and the "miraclee," or the new field my friend Mike called miracology.

NOTES

1. Raymond Moody, *Reflections of Life After Life* (New York: Bantam Books, 1977).
2. George Gallup, Jr., *Adventures in Immortality* (New York: McGraw-Hill, 1982).
3. Arnold Toynbee and Arthur Koestler, eds., *Life After Death* (London: Weldenfeld and Nicolson, 1976), 238–239.
4. Examples of research in NDEs are found in R. L. MacMillan and K. W. G. Brown, "Cardiac Arrest Remembered," *Canadian Medical Association Journal* 104 (1971): 889; and I. Stevenson, "Research into the Evidence of Man's Survival after Death," *Journal of Nervous and Mental Disease* 165, no. 3 (1977): 152–170. See also D. R. Wheeler, *Journey to the Other Side* (New York: Ace Books, 1976) in which several reports from "clinically dead" patients are presented.
5. The "perceptual release" theory was first proposed in 1931 by neurologist J. H. Jackson, *Selected Writings* (London: Hodder and Stoughton, 1931). For a more recent description of this theory, see psychiatrist L. J. West, "A Clinical and Theoretical Overview of Hallucinatory Phenomena," in *Hallucinations: Behavior, Experience, and Theory*, ed. R. K. Siegel and L. J. West (New York: John Wiley, 1975), 287–311.
6. Wilder Penfield, *The Mystery of the Mind* (Princeton, NJ: Princeton University Press, 1975).
7. Michael Sabom, *Recollections of Death* (London: Corgi, 1982), 252.
8. Patrick Gallagher, "Over Easy: A Cultural Anthropologist's Near-Death Experience," *Anabiosis* 2, no. 2 (1982): 140–149.
9. Baruch Spinoza, "Of Miracles," in *The Philosophy of Spinoza* (New York: Random House, 1927).
10. Guy Murchie, *The Seven Mysteries of Life: An Exploration in Science and Philosophy* (Boston: Houghton Mifflin, 1978).
11. Frank Wilczek and Betsy Devine, *Longing for the Harmonies: Themes and Variations from Modern Physics* (New York: W. W. Norton, 1987).
12. J. Allen Hynek, sometimes referred to as America's leading UFOlogist established the UFO hot line (UFO-1000) for around-the-clock reporting of UFOs. His findings and views are reported in J. A. Hynek, "The Emerging Picture of the UFO Problem," *American Institute of Aeronautics and Astronautics* 75, no. 41 (1975).

13. Richard Heinberg, *Memories and Visions of Paradise: Exploring the Universal Myth of a Lost Golden Age* (Los Angeles: Tarcher, 1989), 211–217.

14. Toni Eatts, "Nimbin Spirits," *Sydney Sunday Telegraph*, July 1987, quoted in Heinberg, *Memories and Visions of Paradise*, 216–217.

15. Mircea Eliade, *Shamanism* (Princeton, NJ: Princeton University Press, 1964), 99. For further information and reports about the levitation, spirituality, luminosity of glowing of the human spirit, see also Mircea Eliade, *The Sacred and the Profane* (New York: Harcourt Brace and World, 1959); *Myths, Dreams, and Mysteries* (New York: Harper & Row, 1967); and *Patterns in Comparative Religion* (New York: New American Library, 1974).

16. Quoted in Heinberg, *Memories and Visions of Paradise*, 217.

17. Paul Davies, *God and the New Physics* (New York: Simon & Schuster, 1983), 197.

18. William Irwin Thompson, *Evil and World Order* (New York: Harper & Row, 1976).

19. *Ibid.*, 81.

20. See Arthur Koestler, *The Case of the Midwife Toad* (New York: Random House, 1973). Also Alister Hardie, Robert Harvie, and Arthur Koestler, *The Challenge of Chance* (London: Hutchinson, 1973).

21. Paul Kammerer, *Das Gestex der Serie* (Stuttgart-Berlin: Deutsche Verlags-Ansalt, 1919). See also Arthur Koestler, *The Roots of Coincidence* (New York: Random House, 1972).

22. Kammerer, *Das Geslex der Serie*.

23. Carl Sergeant and Hans Eysenck, *Explaining the Unexplained* (London: Weidenfeld and Nicolson, 1982), 183.

24. J. B. Priestly, *Man and Time* (London: Aldus Books, 1964).

25. Stephen Hawking, *A Brief History of Time* (New York: Bantam Books, 1988), 175.

26. Baruch Spinoza. *The Philosophy of Spinoza*. Introduction by Joseph Ratner (New York: Random House, 1927), 46.

27. William Masters and Virginia Johnson, *Human Sexual Response* (Boston: Little, Brown, 1966).

28. The story as told by Dame Rebecca West is quoted in Michael Shallis, *On Time* (New York: Shocken, 1983), 133.

29. Jeremy W. Hayward, *Shifting Worlds: Changing Minds Where the Sciences and Buddhism Meet* (Boston: Shambhala, 1987), 173.

30. An interesting discussion of the "psychology of flow" is presented by psychologist Mihaly Csikszentmihalyi, *Flow: The Psychology of Optimal Experience* (New York: HarperCollins, 1990). Csikszentmihalyi suggests that mathematical calculation yields the possibility that we process about 126 bits of information per second; 7,560 per minute; or

0.5 million per hour. Over our lifetimes, we process 185 billion bits of information, and too often we are busy fighting and fleeing rather than flowing (matching our dreams, abilities, and opportunities in the direction of our sensed destiny).

31. Hayward, *Shifting Worlds*, 172.

4
BECOMING A MIRACLE MAKER

The "Abnormalcy Advantage"

> What we call "normal" in psychology is really a psycho-
> pathology of the average, so undramatic and so widely
> spread that we don't even notice it.
> —ABRAHAM MASLOW

Patsy's Parade

"I see the balloons!" screamed little Patsy. "I see the balloons!
They're blowing them all up right there for the parade. But that
little balloon won't stay up. It just can't hold air. It can't keep the air
inside it. It must feel like me."

Patsy was a miracle maker. She was only eight years old but she
had wisdom that many don't have even after decades of living. Her
favorite statement was, "That's just the way." All of her games
followed the rules of "the way." She was undergoing a bone marrow
transplant as treatment for her leukemia. She was in the hospital
room next to mine, and on this Thanksgiving morning, her
screams were of excitement and not from the pain of the needles
that usually began our mornings.

Patsy often sat with the nurses at their station. They needed her
to boost their courage on one of the most stress-inducing units of

any hospital. The entire floor is sealed off from the rest of the hospital and has its own air circulation to save us patients from contracting infections. Our immunity was down to zero because of chemotherapy and radiation, and our blood counts would have signaled death under normal circumstances. A common cold could kill dozens of us within days. Masks, gowns, and sterile gloves were worn by everyone, including the limited number of visitors, who always seemed so afraid when they came to see us. Once on this unit, we patients seldom felt the touch of another person's skin against our own. There were many "almost hugs" that stopped short of contact for fear of contamination. We learned to signal our hugging by wrapping our arms around ourselves while our loved ones hugged themselves.

All of us were on the verge of death. Almost half of us would die. Most of us would be exposed to more radiation than the workers in the nuclear accident in Chernobyl. In fact, lessons learned from treating the victims of nuclear accidents were applied to the treatment of bone marrow transplant patients.

We were all in terrible pain, constantly vomiting and losing control of our bowels at the same time. We were sick with repeated infections, and festering oral sores from the chemotherapy grew so large that they almost sealed off our mouths and made swallowing nearly impossible. We were all losing weight and had to be fed through our veins because radiation treatments had burned our appetites away. We ached where needles had drilled into our bones to withdraw marrow samples. I have never known such pain as the sensation of my own marrow being sucked from deep within me.

A bone marrow transplant typically requires about two months of hospitalization in almost total isolation. Prior to this time, the most rigorous tests are conducted and, ironically, the candidates for a transplant must be in "good health" even though they are dying. A "donor transplant" is a process through which the patient receives bone marrow provided by someone who perfectly matches the patient's own. An autologous transplant, as in my case, requires the removal of the patient's own marrow, sometimes "purging" or treating it with intense chemotherapy, and then placing the marrow back inside the body after the patient has had days of near-lethal whole-body radiation and/or chemotherapy. Including the diagnosis, evaluation, numerous tests, chemotherapy and radiation therapy, transfusions, and lengthy recuperation during which the immunity of the patient is so low that every cough and sneeze causes a fear of death, the patient and his or her family surrenders any semblance of a normal life for about two years.

All of us looked like walking ghosts. "I have an idea for a new diet," said Patsy one morning when we all were getting weighed. "Everyone who wants to look skinny can come here to get chemicals and rays. Then they will look like us. They could go on our cancer diet."

We could hear each other retching during the night and crying all day, but Patsy would cry only for a little while. Then she would hop onto her metal stand, which held the IV bags and tubes that always dangled beside each of us. Each stand was hung with several different colored bags that ballooned out in fullness with toxic chemicals designed to burn away any growing cell in our body, the latest drugs to treat the many infections we all contracted, and nutrients to keep us alive while we were unable to eat and digest food. The chemotherapy medications were equal-opportunity killers. They attacked any fast-growing cell in the body, whether or not that cell was a normal hair or stomach-lining cell or a killer cancer cell. The contents stung and destroyed our veins so completely that the multiple daily blood tests we received had to be taken from a plastic catheter surgically implanted in our chests.

In the middle of the night, the nurses would come to pop out the heparin seals that served as chemical corks to hold back the blood in our chest tubes. The blood would spurt out, sometimes soaking the patient, nurse, and bed. Hundreds of blood tests were necessary to determine when transfusions would be needed to save our lives. We sometimes tried to pretend we were not awake when the blood was taken, but the smell of heparin and our own blood would nauseate us. We patients called this catheter the "Dracula Drain," but our feeble attempt at humor could not mask our terror.

When we were given platelets to increase our blood count, we would feel freezing cold. I shook so hard that I still have soreness in my joints and muscles. A sudden fever would result, followed by tremors, headache, and nausea. All of this was overwhelming for a grown man, but Patsy weathered each torturing procedure with humor and strength. Her presence permeated the entire unit.

Patsy loved to ride her IV stand, crouched so low that the nurses saw only what seemed to be an unguided stand moving past their high counter. Patsy sneaked by the nurses' station and rode what she called her Christmas tree IV stand every day, and we all laughed at this daily joke. She would often drag along dolls in her parade and demanded that patients who were out for a wobbly walk join her. We had to keep in line, because that was Patsy's way. The nurses and doctors came to rely on Patsy's procession as a boost to their morale and energy, and we patients came to see her parade as a form of protest against the overwhelming urge to give up.

Now, however, Patsy was losing her physical battle. The transplant had taken just too much from her, and although she had pulled through countless crises that should have killed her, this time she would not survive. A virus so small and so weak that almost any person would never be bothered by it eventually would take advantage of Patsy's lowered immunity and kill her. First, there would be a slight fever and then, within hours, Patsy would be gone. Still, she continued to humble all of us with her strength and the making of her miracles.

On this Thanksgiving morning just before the crisis that all of us feared could happen to any of us at any time, her cries were of excitement about preparations for the Detroit Thanksgiving Day parade that were taking place (by coincidence) right underneath her window in the hospital courtyard. She hollered with glee at the big, multicolored balloons, and we all clustered to Patsy's room, dragging our own Christmas tree IVs. Like prisoners pressed up against the bars of our cell, we looked down on the impending holiday celebration.

"But that one little balloon can't hold air," said Patsy. She had been unusually pensive the last several days, and we all noticed that Patsy's parade was not taking place as regularly as it once did. She became somber now as she pressed her nose to the hospital window. We pretended we could not hear her murmur, "That's just the way."

Suddenly, the little balloon inflated and floated away from its handler and up into the sky. "There it goes" yelled Patsy. "It's going to heaven, but the parade is still going to go on, isn't it? There are lots of balloons and air is everywhere. That's the way it will be."

With her words, the little balloon's journey seemed to be a meaningful coincidence for Patsy and for us all.

The Timelessness of Miracles

After my own bone marrow transplant, I almost died from suffocation. A simple virus not unlike the one that took Patsy's life attacked my lungs. As the nurses rushed me to surgery and I gasped for air, my nurse Carolyn said, "Remember Patsy and her parades. Think of your lungs as balloons and try to fill them up with air. Find the way." That's all she said, but it was all she had to say. She knew I needed Patsy's spirit then. I could barely breathe, but I relaxed as I felt comfort in Patsy's principle of "the way."

I survived what was supposed to be an "always fatal virus" to bone marrow transplant patients, and I began to breathe again. I had been given strength from Patsy. I knew her to be a miracle maker. I knew her spirit was still making miracles for all of us. Patsy had not survived her own illness, but miracles are not measured individually and in linear time. The measure of miracles is not living to an old age but of living life with the confidence that there is much more to life than just a local living. Miracles are not measured as successes but as celebrations of the strength and eternity of the human spirit.

The healing energy of Patsy's living provides clues for what it takes to be a miracle maker. Patsy's life must be measured in the depth and meaning she brought to it, not in the number of her years and birthdays. The science principles of nonlocality and nonlinearity are proven through the power, pervasiveness, and permanence of who Patsy always will be. Patsy lives forever in her enduring relationship with all of us. The temple of miracles is in our relationships and in our connectedness to others, not in our body or our skills. I will never see a balloon or a parade without feeling Patsy's power.

If we use long life, heroic survival, and the conquering of disease as the exclusive criteria of a miracle, we are trapped into believing that miracles "happen" only to a chosen few. We seem to think that if we are very lucky, very good, or try very hard, a miracle will happen "to" us and we will achieve victory over time, space, disease, and grief. But miracles are not payoffs for earned cosmic points. Miracles occur when we perceive life from the perspective of the cosmic laws or the "way it is" in the universe.

If we are impressed only by the misguided miracles of levitation or by dramatic stories of heroic patients conquering disease, we fail to see the simple miracles of a cloud moving at just the right time, a silver lunar rainbow, or the glory of a Christmas tree IV protest parade in support of healing. We can copy and learn from miracle makers such as Patsy. They know how to do everyday miracles.

Miracle makers like Patsy have found the way. As philosopher Sengtsan writes, "For the unified mind in accord with the Way all self-centered striving ceases."[1] In other words, miracles have little to do with the survival of the self unless that self is all of us. Miracle makers are aware of their nonlocality, as when Patsy saw herself as one with the little balloon that escaped the confines of earth. They know that their chosen view of their world designs that world, as when Patsy made joyful parades in a place where funeral processions were more likely. They know of the principle of complementarity, as when Patsy saw our potential for marching in her parade even as we wobbled down the hospital hall. They know the hope that comes with the uncertainty of life, as Patsy seemed to know when she pensively looked out of her hospital window and said that the parade would always go on even though some balloons escaped. After twenty-five years of clinical work with my seventeen miracle makers and after my own near-death experiences, I now know that we don't have to go to gurus or channelers to find our role models for miracle making; we just have to look for people like Patsy.

Spiritual Superstars

An elitism of miracles has evolved in recent years. Popular and scientific writers alike describe the "heroic patient who conquers a fatal disease" and gurus who have uncommon insight and clearness of thought. There is talk of channelers, precognizers, fortune-tellers, and mystics who are able to see what the rest of us cannot.

My professional and personal experiences have taught me that although some people may indeed have developed their God-given capacity for uncommon consciousness, they are only professional spiritual athletes. The true gurus are common people who are able to cluster coincidences around them and give them meaning. They are free from the constraints of a local, time-limited view of the world, but they have *not* surrendered their rationality in achieving that freedom.

The Common Consciousness Cosmonauts

Brendan O'Regan, vice-president for research at the Institute of Noetic Science in Sausalito, California, is analyzing data on miracles that are reported all over the world. He has visited Lourdes in France and Medjugore in Yugoslavia, where an apparition of the Virgin Mary appeared in 1981. He has reviewed more than 860 medical journals and more than 3,000 individual articles on "spontaneous cures" and "coincidental remissions."[2] His detailed analysis establishes the legitimacy and commonness of miracles.

Father Slavko, a Franciscan monk who holds a Ph.D. in psychology and lives and works at the shrine at Medjugore, has noticed common characteristics in those people who are healed by their experience of going there. O'Regan writes, "It's very often the people who come and don't determinedly want healing who are affected. They come with an open mind and ask for healing but they have not come with this as the single-minded purpose of their trip."[3]

My own experience working with my patients supports this "openness to the Way" orientation of the miracle makers. Just as it is not the library that causes us to learn, so it is not the shrines at Medjugore or Lourdes that provide the miracle. Miracle makers go to shrines for a place to do, not find, their miracle. *It is not determination toward a specific goal, but rather acceptance of cosmic life laws and a desire to experience all sides of living to its fullest* that sets the stage for miracle making.

The Home on the Range Approach

"You always seem to look so pensive," said Marjorie. She was the always-cheerful nurse who seemed to believe in what I called the "home on the range" approach to illness and healing. The famous song titled "Home on the Range" contains the phrase "where seldom is heard a discouraging word and the skies are not cloudy all day."

Although Marjorie's optimism was sincere, too often some people practice a pseudopsychology of mind-over-matter healing that suggests that we be upbeat, courageous, and maintain a positive attitude at all times. While there is nothing wrong with cheerfulness, I have found reflection, yearning, and private searching for life's meaning also to be key steps in the making of miracles. Crying in awe of the endurance of the human spirit is as healing as laughing in hope.

Suffering increases the potential for meaningful miracles because suffering increases our awareness of the nonlocality of the self. The suffering of cancer and its related treatments forced my attention away from "me" and toward a deep reflection on the nature of life and its meaning, a sense of my connection with everyone and everything, and direct, personal experience of the "Way" things are.

In his study of those who have made their own miracles, psychologist Brendan O'Regan did not see the ever-happy and cheerful orientation of popular psychology. He writes, "There is a sad, faraway look in their eyes . . . that is unmistakable. It seems like a kind of yearning for something, the search for a memory."[4] O'Regan may have mistaken for sadness a contemplative state that I have seen in the miracle makers whom I have studied. The yearning of the miracle maker is a yearning for the finding of the Way. Perhaps the "farawayness" in their eyes was evidence of their realization of their nonlocality and the fact that none of us are trapped "here." The memory for which O'Regan's patients seem to be searching may be our collective capacity to transcend our physical state and to put our spirits to work in the making of our miracles.

Aldous Huxley wrote, "The capacity to suffer arises where there is imperfection, disunity, and separation from an embracing totality."[5] A key step in making miracles is to be aware of how much more you are than just a body in a specific moment and place. Instead of being home on the range, miracles are found by working toward an awareness of our true nature as being everywhere.

Vittorio Micheli Went for a Walk

Miracologist and researcher O'Regan describes a case similar to my own.[6] He discusses an event that happened in May 1962 involving a middle-aged Italian man with a large tumor in his left pelvic area. (My soccer-ball–size tumor was in the right side of my pelvis.) O'Regan reports that the tumor was so massive that it ate away this man's left hip and left him in excruciating pain. (My tumor ate away my right hip and the pain I experienced was immense and totally debilitating.) As in my case, a biopsy showed that the tumor was an aggressive, usually fatal, form of cancer.

For some reason, the man did not receive treatments for ten months. I was misdiagnosed for eight months, and in both of our cases, our skeletons were being destroyed. The man went to Lourdes, where he was bathed. Reports from the Medical Commission of Lourdes record that, exactly as I experienced, the man had lost significant amounts of weight, was in constant pain, and was unable to eat.

After his return from Lourdes, according to O'Regan's report, Mr. Micheli began to regain his appetite and noticed more mobility in his legs. About one month later, doctors took X rays. The man's cancer, as in my case, had decreased significantly in size. Then, in May 1963, the tumor disappeared and, as reported by physician Larry Dossey, "Another event happened that was even more amazing than the disappearance of the tumor. The bone of the pelvis, hip, and femur began to regrow, and with time completely reconstructed itself! Two months after being bathed at Lourdes, Vittorio Micheli went for a walk."[7]

The physician's report of Mr. Micheli's case read, in part, "The X rays confirm categorically and without doubt that an unforeseen and even overwhelming bone reconstruction has taken place of a type unknown in the annals of world medicine. The patient is alive and in a flourishing state of health nine years after his return from Lourdes."[8]

My own report reads, "Dr. Pearsall has experienced a miraculous cure. His prognosis is excellent." My X rays had to be repeated because the radiologists could not be convinced that my current films were truly my own. "There has been a terrible mistake," one doctor said to me. "We lost your X rays and we have the wrong set. This man's bones are fully intact." Repeat X rays confirmed the miracle. Vittorio and I lived a very similar miracle.

I did not go to Lourdes, but I did go to my family and to my healing place in Maui. I employed several assistant miracle makers from the ranks of doctors and nurses. My nurses Carolyn, Marjorie, Betsy, and others never let *local* problems determine my fate. They never yielded to the *certainty* that can convert a diagnosis to a verdict, and they never allowed the limited point of view of an expert *observer* to determine the course of my healing or prevent them from helping to save my life in any way they could. The skilled and creative team of doctors on the Bone Marrow Transplant Team at Harper Hospital of Detroit (part of the Wayne State University Medical Center) were always open to the *complementary* side of every medical option. While they battled my disease on a "particle" level, my little "medicine girl" Patsy, my family, and the other courageous patients on my transplant unit kept me connected with the life-saving "waves" of love. Miracles are always an "us" thing, and miracle makers are very good at making nonlocal, spiritual connections with people (I will examine the loving nature of the miracle maker in more detail in chapter 5). Every day, there are miracles in families who manage to give their impaired children joyful lives, who survive the ravages of substance abuse, and who hold together as individuals and as a family through the most trying times. Miracles are not reserved for heroic "survivors." Miracles are made when people live life with meaning and satisfaction, even when negative circumstances surround them.

The Midas Mistake and the Danger of Making Wishes

Miracle making has nothing to do with making wishes. People who make wishes are taking a dangerous risk. As in fairy tales, most of our wishes come true. Unfortunately, we usually regret getting what we wished for because our wishes ultimately contradict the principles of the cosmos. We make the mistake of wishing for "our" way instead of the Way of Patsy's principle.

We tend to make what I call the "Midas Mistake." King Midas wished that everything he touched be turned to gold. He got his wish, and with it he lost forever the warmth and loving he really needed as those around him turned to cold, unresponsive gold metal. The miracle he wished for ultimately isolated and destroyed him and all those around him.

If we wish for miracles, we not only fail to exercise our own miracle-making capabilities but we are trying to assume the impossible position of a nonparticipant observer who is asking the world to change around, but not because of, us. Moreover, we run the risk of suffering from the attainment of our wish, because our certainty about how our world "should" be conflicts with the uncertainty principle that rules the cosmos. Wishing implies that having all of something is better than having a complementary balance in living. This conviction violates the complementarity principle. Miracle making involves the active embracing of the Way of our spiritual life, but it does not imply an acquiescent, helpless view of living. The act of wishing, in contrast, suggests a passive role rather than the participatory observer role so basic to the laws of the cosmos. Wishing denotes a request for intervention from "without," which violates the law of nonlocality that emphasizes the unity of everything and everyone. Miracle making represents a discovery of a new way of knowing from "within." If wishing is *longing* for love, then miracle making is active *loving* through every crisis and challenge in daily living.

If you wish for perfect health forever, you will never know what perfect health really is because you will never know the complementary side of health, which is illness. If you wish for perfect love with no conflict in your relationships, you will never value fully the miracle of being loved because you have never known the pain of its loss. Wished-for love is a passive love; love attained is an active, volitional state. Just as miracles do not happen to us, love does not happen to us. We make love by doing it, showing it, and realizing that, like illness is a part of health, so hurt and loss are a part of loving. Finally, if you wish for immortality, you will not share the full journey of life with those you love. You will end up always being the person losing other persons and never be the person who is lost.

When I teach about the art of miracle making, I ask my patients and students to ask themselves the following question: If you could have just one wish and be guaranteed that your wish would come true, what would that wish be? No matter what they answer, I ask them to consider the principle of complementarity: What about the exact opposite of your wish? Might that not make you equally happy in a different way? Are you really so certain about your wish?

If you wish for wealth, for example, would you not be as happy with simplicity? If your wish were granted, would you truly be happy with the complexities and obligations that come with wealth? If you wish for health, would you ever want to know what everyone else will know and learn from their times of sickness and suffering; will you miss the blessed feeling of renewed energy, the resumption of living, and the spiritual introspection that come with illness? Would you want to be the only one among your friends and loved ones who was healthy, unable to understand others' suffering?

We humans tend to think that if a little bit of something is nice, even more would be better.[9] This is the local, one-cause-equals-one-effect, linear view of the world. Actually, the laws of physics teach that a little bit of something is just enough so long as we remember the complementary side of everything we think we want or need. That is why miracle makers are not wishers for more; they are readers of what is. They are active and participating observers of their own lives and the lives of those around them.

Becoming Miracle Prone

Based on my own experiences with miracles,[10] my clinical study of meaningful coincidences and of seventeen patients who beat the odds by not allowing a diagnosis of death to be a wrongful verdict of nothingness, and research by others in this most exciting of human adventures, I have identified six characteristics of people who are what I call miracle prone. These are

- A confident, erect posture with eyes that convey a spiritual energy and a *knowing* beyond the rational, logical, simplistic knowing of everyday living. They seem to know that their role of *observer* is crucial to what they will see.
- Experience with several crises, and in the process, the development of a *psychic toughness,* as well as an awareness that there is always a *complementary* side to even the most apparently hopeless situation.
- A *yearning* for much more from life than mere coping, survival, success, and security. A desire to behave in ways compatible with our *nonlocality* or transcendence of the here and now.
- A *simplicity* of lifestyle free of the need to acquire goods and possess expensive, complex things.

- An *abnormal* attitude in the sense that they are creative and have avoided becoming "well adjusted" to a linear, stressful, see-and-touch world.
- A tendency to be *psychic gamblers* because they are willing to take risks for the fulfillment of their dreams and to give meaning to the signals sent by the coincidences in their lives. They think in a freewheeling style that reflects the *uncertainty* of all of life.

The remainder of this chapter will explore each of these characteristics in greater detail. I invite you to learn the skill of miracle making from this list, for it is a skill that most certainly will make your life much more lively—and may even save your life, as it did mine.

The Look of the Lucky

As Brendan O'Regan writes, people who experience miracles "are in a very different place psychologically, emotionally, and indeed psychophysiologically."[11] Most miracle makers resemble this description by an oncology nurse who treated me:

Every one of the patients who made it happen, who made miracles, looked the same. It was in their eyes, their posture, their hands, and their body. They had a dreamy look, like they were somewhere else other than here getting their treatments. I even had to tell them when the treatment was over. It was like I had to bring them back to earth. They also had what I call gentle moving hands. They touched softly, easily, and gently. Maybe it was because they were all weak, but I think they touched like that naturally. They all stood upright, as if their body was being held up by something other than muscles and bones. And I know this sounds terrible, but they all seemed to be skinny. Not because they had lost weight or were sick. They were on the trim side, each one of them. That's it. Dreamy, skinny, gentle, and upright.[12]

I make no claim that my seventeen MMs are scientifically representative of a "type" of person. I am sure, however, that they and I were physically altered by the impact of a life orientation. I believe that miracle makers look "dreamy" because they experience the nonlocality of our existence. They look dreamy because they have a dream that transcends the here and now.

The energy expended in making miracles can burn off calories just like any other form of exercise. If there is sometimes a gaunt, drawn look to miracle makers, it may be due to their constant energetic exchange with everyone and everything. These are players in the major leagues of our nonlocality.

Miracle makers move and touch gently because in many ways they are just barely in their own body. Movements are made of necessity, but the soul is of the essence.

I believe that miracle makers stand tall because they are buttressed by their awareness of the glory of it all; their appreciation of the unrestricted, unlimited, immortal human spirit. Their bodies are not just held up by muscle and bone. They are buoyed in the often turbulent sea of daily living by their cosmic connection.

There are many plausible explanations for this "look of the lucky." Perhaps poor appetite, fear, depression, helplessness, and side effects of their many physical problems contribute more significantly to the look than their choice of a nonlocal view of living. That is the traditional, easy, local view. I choose the more radical, nonlocal view. I hope you will make the same choice.

The Psychic Toughness Response

There have been numerous books and articles about the fight-or-flight response, the sexual response, and the relaxation response. Recent research suggests that there is also a "toughness response," a training of the body and mind to better tolerate the neurochemical effects of stress through constant stress exercise. Just as someone lifts weights to develop physical strength, so the person with psychic toughness has carried many heavy loads, thereby conditioning themselves through their minicrises. As a result, their psychophysiological strength and adaptability develops to a higher level of psychic fitness.[13]

When working with paraplegic men and women, I noticed that they typically showed this psychic toughness response. Perhaps because paraplegic persons are unable to use their bodies to cope with some challenges, they must develop a sharper mental toughness. They can lose their temper and get upset without paying the price that less-tough individuals pay when the killer stress chemicals shoot through the body, stimulating it to fight or flee.

The MMs all showed a psychic toughness. They had dealt with several stressors in their life before their present severe crises and had heightened coping capacity. In the film *Lawrence of Arabia*, T. E. Lawrence performs a minor miracle. He holds his hand over a candle flame until his flesh starts to cook. When his friend tries this same trick, he screams in pain as he pulls away. He asks Lawrence if the flame did not hurt his hand. Lawrence answers, "Yes, but the trick is not to mind."

Like magicians mastering sleight of hand, the MMs all had learned the skill that I call sleight of mind. They had become psychically toughened by a series of pain and suffering, and they had learned not to react only with their body. Thus they functioned within the realm of nonlocality, dispersing their pain rather than focusing on it as an exclusive somatic experience.

I have attempted to describe the pain of my illness and treatments throughout this book. I have found the task to be impossible. In her essay "On Being Ill," author Virginia Woolf writes that our language can express the images of Hamlet and the tragedy of Lear, but "try to describe a pain . . . to a doctor and language at once runs dry."[14] The description of pain eludes us because pain is such a subjective event. Because it is subjective, we ourselves give it most of its power and meaning.

When we have been forced to cope with severe pain many times, we learn a sleight of mind to prevent pain from overwhelming us. The miracle maker converts severe pain to an energy to escape local suffering to the safety of other realms of reality. If we have developed a psychological toughness, severe pain drives us from our body and into our souls.

A friend of mine asked me how I could possibly deal with a diagnosis of death and all of the related suffering of my disease. I answered, "Just like other people in my situation, this is not the first problem in my life. My wife and I struggled through painful tests to 'confirm' a diagnosis of infertility, only to have our own biological child years later. We now have one son with cerebral palsy and another with a severe learning disability and dyslexia. My wife and I have seen our fathers die suddenly. I have had six surgeries and faced the possibility of blindness twice because of

retinal detachments. We've been here before. We call it our agony
aerobics. I think we've built up a torture tolerance."

My friend laughed, but I was serious. I believe that we can
develop spiritual stamina. Following the principle of complementarity, crises complement healing. Miracle makers use their problems to make themselves stronger. We learn to make miracles out
of madness when we get used to dealing with madness on a
regular basis.

If your own life seems problem prone, you are in forced training
for miracle making. Your choice is whether to view the apparent
unfairness of so many problems happening to one person or
family as victimization or as a painful part of learning to make
miracles.

Yearning for More

Miracle makers are actively engaged in a search for the meaning of
life. No coincidence is a "simple" coincidence to the miracle maker.
As one MM said, "Everything means something." Something inside the MM knows that there are many ways to know, and so the
miracle maker is locked in the pursuit of a meaning to life that
extends far beyond success and survival.

Two unusual words describe the focus of the miracle maker:
ineffability and *noesis.* Ineffability refers to an experience of our
nonlocality of such power, so different from the sense-oriented,
local view of life that it almost defies description. "I can't say it or
tell it," said eight-year-old Patsy, the little miracle maker on the
bone marrow transplant unit. "It's really strange at night when you
think you have a new bone marrow but you don't have a new you.
Where are you and who are you? I don't know. I mean I think I
know, but I can't tell it."

Patsy spoke in metaphors when she spoke of the balloon that
broke away. Religious figures, prophets, and wise people often
speak in parables, analogies, or riddles because they are trying to
describe things that are indescribable using our ordinary vocabulary. Illustrating meaning through metaphor is one way to communicate the ineffable.

Noesis refers to the sense of heightened clarity and nonlocality
that miracle makers experience. Early works refer to such knowing

as "cosmic consciousness"[15] or "peak experiences."[16] Psychologist Roger Walsh writes of this reality as being "so discordant with our usual picture of reality, so paradoxical, as to defy description in traditional terms and theories and to call into question some of the most fundamental assumptions of Western science and philosophy."[17]

If you choose to be a miracle maker, another choice you will have to make is whether or not you are willing to embark on a search for the meaning of the cosmic occurrences and meaningful miracles that show our human spirit in action.

We must, of course, earn our living, raise our children, and survive in the whirlwind of obligations of daily life. We must do what is necessary to adapt to the see-and-touch world, but we must realize that no matter how much we are "doing," we can still contemplate our "being" and our purpose for being. Like everyone else, I spend time balancing my checkbook, paying my taxes, going to the dentist, cleaning the house, and fixing the car. Even as I do what is necessary, however, the principle of complementarity causes me to think of how close I have come to not being able to do anything again. I think about what is truly miraculous about being alive and ponder *why* I am doing what I am doing. I can remember my dreams and monitor my life for its fit with those dreams. Am I loving enough, working at what I choose to work at, writing books I believe in, reading what I would like to read, and spending time with my loved ones? Am I remembering my connection with everyone, my responsibilities to the world ecology and to the welfare of others, and the fact that I must never stop yearning for the miracle of peace, harmony, and sharing? Whenever I start to feel too content, I know that such satisfaction stems from the see-and-touch world's seduction with doing rather than the miracle of our being.

Freedom from "Stuff-itis"

When you face death, one of the first things you learn is how unimportant "stuff" is. One of my seventeen MMs, a biophysicist who recently died of cancer, had created many of his own miracles before and during his illness. He had outlived the most dire predictions about his condition. He said,

I used to be a molecule collector. I was into getting more and more particles. Now, I'm a meaning collector. I'm into getting more and more waves, more and more energy in my life; more spirit and less stuff. My wife and I had so much stuff that we graduated to the postgraduate level of garage sale shopping: We found ourselves going to garage sales to find holders for the stuff that we bought at other garage sales! Now, I want to spend my time without stuff all around me. I want to feel sun and wind, the rain, the night. I want to feel myself thinking and feeling. I don't want stuff—getting stuff, finding and protecting and maintaining stuff—to get in the way anymore. I want to live my life, not spend it sorting through the clutter that really has nothing to do with living.

We live in Michigan during the summer, and my wife set up a hospital room in our home there during my first chemotherapy. As I lay in a hospital bed in the family room, I watched my neighbor trimming the large bushes around his swimming pool. My neighbor started in early spring and swore all summer long as he cut at the bushes he had planted there and the bushes cut him back. He saw no relationship between himself and the natural vegetation, which had become invading stuff that detracted from his more important stuff, such as his pool and walls of his house. I never saw him admire his landscaping as he struggled to control it. He found no joy in his yard, but at the end of the summer, I saw him bring home more than a dozen new bushes to fight with next spring. I promised myself that day that if I was given more time to live I would attend more to *relating with* instead of *working on* my world.

I have learned to take time to look at my yard at least as often as I work in it. Until I was forced by my illness to take the time to look, I never noticed how much time we spend maintaining rather than enjoying our life. Now, when I cut my lawn or prune my bushes, I copy my Maui gardener, Pete, who always pauses to smell, talk to, touch, and look at the natural beauty around him. For the first time, I have seen where I live instead of rushing through my world. Now, when I walk around my yard, I can feel the bushes, lawn, and flowers rather than see them as potential chores. They continue to cure me by their very presence, and I sense the miracle in the existence they share with me.

A key choice in learning to make miracles is deciding whether or not you will be a consumer or be consumed. There is little time for miracle making when you are busy fixing, repairing, maintaining, and getting.

Comedienne Irma Bombeck wrote, "Never buy anything that eats or needs repairing."[18] This philosophy of simplicity can clear the way for more meaningful living. During one of the most dreadful moments of his illness, a young bank executive MM said, "I've done, gotten, broken, and fixed almost everything, but I don't remember living."

We all must take care of the place we live, buy clothes to wear, and keep some order in our lives. If we are to make miracles, however, we must remember that the stuff of our lives are only the necessary facilitators for our movement within our physical world, not objectives in themselves.

When I went into the hospital for my bone marrow transplant, the nurses told me that I could bring everything I needed. "You'll be living here for months, so bring what you need," said one nurse. I knew I would be busy trying to make miracles, so I wondered what I would really need to do so. What stuff would you take along for miracle making?

For me, the choice was easy. I took plenty of paper and pens. I asked several of my family and friends to buy me books that they were sure I would not read. I asked for books I would never buy for myself. I was hoping that I could create some meaningful coincidences by this merging of paper, pen, and new ideas. My wife bought me a book titled *What Are the Chances?* by Bernard Siskin and Jerome Staller. It's a thin book with nothing but statistical chances listed throughout.

One day, as I suffered through some particularly painful chemotherapy and was wondering how I could have come down with cancer when no one in my family had ever had it and I never smoked and had followed almost every healthcare warning, I grabbed the book my wife had given me, thinking that its lack of plot and simple listing of interesting facts would distract me. I randomly opened the book to the middle and read, "Radiological studies of the gastrointestinal tract . . . are 90 times [the radiation] that you are exposed to during a typical dental X-ray."[19]

Over the last fifteen years, I had received dozens of X rays of the abdominal area as part of the diagnosis and treatment of kidney stones, and I mentioned this at once to my doctors. They now tell me that it is possible that these powerful X rays may have contributed to my developing cancer. By coincidence, a meaningful clue to the etiology of my disease had been revealed, as well as a clue for preventing its recurrence by avoiding X rays as much as possible. A meaningful coincidence had taken place that would direct my healthcare.

The Energy of Insight and the Challenge of Change

As a therapist, I have noticed that meaningful coincidences happen very often to my patients just at a key time of transition in their life, when they are confronting a particularly difficult decision or choice, or when they are on the verge of a meaningful insight regarding their life situation. As psychologist Carl Jung suspected, it seems as if the therapist and the patient were able to tap into their collective unconscious, mobilizing the energy involved in significant synchronous events.[20]

This phenomenon of patient-therapist miracle making is confirmed by Swiss analyst and physicist Arnold Mindel.[21] Award-winning physicist Werner Heisenberg (founder of the uncertainty principle) was impressed by Mindel's work and supported Mindel's conclusion that an enormous amount of energy is released at key times in our lives, explaining why synchronicities often occur around birthdays, deaths, falling in love, during important periods in psychotherapy, intense creative work, a change in profession, or serious illness and healing.[22]

Arnold Mindel gives the example of a mentally disturbed patient who claimed that he was Jesus, the creator and destroyer of light. At that very moment, a lighting fixture dropped from the ceiling, knocking the man unconscious.[23] Therapist friends of mine describe similar coincidences taking place when there "seems to be a lot of changing energy going on." To make miracles, we must choose to make change happen, and as psychiatrist Scott Peck suggests, intentionally take the road less traveled. Peck writes, "Problems call forth our courage and our wisdom; indeed they create our courage and our wisdom. It is only because of problems that we grow mentally and spiritually."[24]

Benjamin Franklin wrote, "Those things that hurt, instruct."[25]

When we choose change and make the effort to grow and become, we hurt. When we hurt, as from cancer, grief, or lost love, there is always the possibility of meaningful change in our view of our life. When we hurt and make transitions, meaningful coincidences and miracles take place. Miracle makers have chosen not to take the easy, "normal," well-adjusted road. They have chosen to create their own emergencies of spiritual growth and to take part in the wonderful events that happen when the energy of an evolving spirit is set free.

Taking the Gamble of Creativity

As pointed out earlier, most of the major discoveries of our world are related to meaningful coincidences. One of the primary characteristics of miracle makers is their constant surveillance for coincidences in their lives and their willingness to take the gamble of following the lead of a miracle.

When we coincidentally discover a picture of a relative whom we have not seen for years, we may choose to look at it briefly and put it away, or we may "gamble" by giving meaning to the coincidence and trying to make contact with that relative immediately. One MM said, "I was cleaning our basement and found an old toy my sister and I had played with years and years ago. I was going to just throw it away and keep cleaning, but instead I stopped working, went to the phone, and called her long distance. When she answered the phone, she was crying. She said 'I was just feeling so lonely. Your call came at just the right time.' " The MM's gamble paid off.

One of the most creative men of the last century was Buckminster Fuller. He wrote, "None of us is a genius. Some of us are just less damaged than most."[26] He meant that some of us manage to escape the confines of traditional education, which stresses compliance and achievement at the price of creativity. If you want to make your own miracles, you might learn from the miracle makers and become a coincidence gambler.

Jungians, those therapists who follow the research and writing of psychologist Carl Jung, refer to the "Gambler Syndrome." The Jungian gambler is a person who is willing to risk everything on the metaphorical turn of a given card in the game of life. Such major chance taking is sometimes necessary when the stakes are high, such as times of decision regarding a major medical treatment or the choice of someone to love for life.

"More than 40 percent of patients such as yourself who get a bone marrow transplant do not survive the procedure, the X rays, and the chemotherapy. We cannot tell you what to do. The decision is yours," said Dr. Lyle Sennsenbrenner, leader of the bone marrow transplant team at Harper Hospital. He is a robust man with a mustache that makes him look like one of the captains of the charter boats in Maui's Maalaea Bay. My wife says that he is of average height, but—probably because he helped save my life and because I was always in a wheelchair or hospital bed looking up at him for hope—I remember him as a giant of a man. On this occasion, he explained to my wife and me all of the details relating to one of the most dramatic treatments for cancer in modern medicine: the bone marrow transplant with its whole-body radiation and an almost totally destructive form of chemotherapy.

My wife and I decided to go ahead with the treatment. When we returned for my final preparation, however, the nurse said, "I'm sorry, but before we can proceed, Dr. Sennsenbrenner wants to talk to you and your wife. He'll see you after lunch."

I said, "Something is wrong, isn't it? We are not going to be able to do this one thing that can save my life?"

The nurse answered, "You'll have to talk with Dr. Sennsenbrenner."

That nonanswer was answer enough. After the agony of deciding whether or not to undergo a lifesaving procedure that could kill me, something was going to exclude me from the procedure.

My wife and I sat with our lunch untouched. We cried again as everything seemed to be coming down on us at once. I thought, "Psychic toughness is one thing, but this has got to be overtraining." Our lunch hour seemed more like a year. It ended with us sitting miserably in Dr. Sennsenbrenner's office.

As always, Dr. Sennsenbrenner rushed into his office. He sat down at a table with his nurse, my wife, and I. "I'm afraid there may be something wrong with your bone marrow. A bone marrow transplant will be more difficult now. We'll have to treat your marrow, too, so the risks are all increased."

"You won't tell me what you think my chances are, will you?" I asked him. "I gave you the statistics." he answered. "Since we'll have to purge your marrow, you probably have much less than a fifty-fifty chance of surviving the transplant and its aftermath. Without the procedure, you will likely not survive for long, but most of your last months would not be as terrible as some of the transplant procedure side-effects will be. I'm sorry, but, of course, it's your decision," he answered.

I felt like a gambler about to turn over the one card that either would total twenty-one or cause me to lose everything and suffer dreadfully in the process. In that instant, I felt a severe shot of pain through my hips, where my cancer was. My wife asked, "What's wrong? You must have jumped a foot in the air. You almost levitated right up to the ceiling!"

"Just a reminder, I guess," I answered, knowing now that I would gamble everything to be given the chance to live. I took that chance. The fact that my own marrow was treated for cancer did put me in much more jeopardy. There was now the chance that my marrow would not survive the purging and lay dead in its storage container in the basement of the hospital while my body starved to death for the cells that only marrow can produce. Now, both my marrow and I would have to undergo treatment separately and hope that we would be safely reunited before one or the other of us was killed by our treatment. That one major gamble is partly responsible for the fact that all of my cancer is gone.

At home, before my hospitalization for the transplant and while waiting for the nine-inch wound left by exploratory surgery to heal, I was filing away my lecture material and preparing to take the risk of my life. As I shuffled things around, a piece of paper floated to the floor. I picked it up and read it. It was a quote by Robert Louis Stevenson that I had written down for future lectures. It read, "Life is not a matter of holding good cards, but of playing a poor hand well."[27] I was ready to play the game to the fullest.

The seventeen MMs were all gamblers in the sense described here. One young woman reported, "I just wasn't sure about loving him. I mean, he seemed to be the one for me, but it was going to be a big risk. He was not divorced yet, he was older than I, and he came from a totally different educational and religious background. I was sitting there looking at his picture and eating peanuts. I was throwing them high in the air and trying to catch them in my mouth. They kept hitting me in the eye and on the forehead. Then, for some reason, I decided that if that next peanut goes in my mouth, I'm going to go for it. I'm going to get serious about him. I threw the next peanut higher than any other, and it seemed to hover in the air trying to make up its mind. It was a direct hit. We're happily married now. It's a lucky thing that peanut hit the target."

This story may sound strange, and it may seem to be poor judgment to base a romantic decision on hand and mouth coordination. But like this woman, all of the MMs were gamblers who used coincidence as part of the process of their decision making. This woman fully acknowledged all of the other key variables that go into lasting love, but her decision to work at loving revolved around one key "card" in the game of her life.

Miracle makers often take such risks because they trust that there is something inside them that seems to guide them in the right direction. They also trust their ability to judge the significance of the clues provided by synchronicity and coincidence. They place their bets, but they are sure that *they* are the ones who provide the energy for the spin of the wheel.

Miracle Making as a Common Human Trait

Author Joseph Priestly, whose collection of miracles I referred to earlier, wrote, "There is nothing supernormal and miraculous about this larger temporal freedom of the dreaming self. It is not a privilege enjoyed by a few very strange and special people. It is a part of our common human lot."[28]

I have presented six of the basic characteristics of miracle makers. Each characteristic represents a choice you must make about your own laws of living before you will be able to claim your birthright as a miracle maker:

- You must choose between being creative, open, and vulnerable to the unpredictable energy of spiritual growth or accepting the more predictable local life of the here and now (principle of nonlocality).
- You must choose between accepting transitional life crises as psychic toughening exercises and a necessary part of attend-

ing soul school here on earth or viewing the transitions and tragedies of daily living as punishment or as proof of the bumper sticker axiom that reads "Life's a bitch and then you die" (principle of complementarity).

- You must choose between pursuing your yearning for a spiritual life that connects you with everyone and everything and being teased by a sense that there is more to life than your local existence or immersing yourself in the more known quantities of local laws: immediate pain, periodic pleasure, and easy and quick closure when decisions and problems arise (uncertainty principle).

- You must choose between a view of life that emphasizes simplicity: freedom from acquiring things, goods, and money, or an outlook on life that stresses doing and getting more and more until the things of your life become the focus of your living (observer participantcy).

- You must choose to utilize as a source of learning the energy released at times of personal decision and development, challenges, changes, and transitions of your life rather than adopt the view that things happen randomly to us and have little meaning other than as aggravations and threats to our survival and happiness (principle of nonlocality).

- Most of all, if you are to make your own miracles, you must choose to be a gambler. You must not be foolhardy or reckless, but you must be vigilant for those times when all of the cards are on the table and it is time, as the saying goes, "to know when to hold them, and know when to fold them." You might at first choose to hold and play your cards by taking small chances that follow your spiritual sense and playing when others would decide to leave the game or watch others play. You must choose to put yourself in the miracle position, opening the way for the coincidence clusters that fuel miracles (observer participantcy).

There is, finally, a seventh characteristic of miracle makers and a seventh choice in the making of miracles for the next chapter. Miracle makers have chosen to show a patience, forgiveness, generosity, truthfulness, and equanimity that I call "loving kindness." Every one of the seventeen miracle-making patients whom I studied showed loving kindness in all that they did. This seemed to be the catalyst for the explosion of a meaningful miracle in their life. As we will discover in the next chapter, they had each learned the six sacred secrets of the science of loving.

NOTES

1. Sengtsan, *Verses on the Faith Mind*, trans. E. R. Clarke (Sharon Springs, NY: Zen Center, 1975).
2. Brendan O'Regan, "Healing, Remission, and Miracle Cures," *Institute of Noetic Sciences Special Report* (May 1987): 3–14.
3. *Ibid.*, 11.
4. *Ibid.*, 11.
5. Aldous Huxley, *The Perennial Philosophy* (New York: Harper & Row, 1944), 227.
6. O'Regan, "Healing, Remission, and Miracle Cures," 9.
7. Larry Dossey, *Recovering the Soul: A Scientific and Spiritual Search* (New York: Bantam Books, 1990), 76.
8. O'Regan, "Healing, Remission, and Miracle Cures," 9.
9. In his book *Recovering the Soul*, physician Larry Dossey writes that the wish for the ultimate source of energy has resulted in the crises at Chernobyl and Three-Mile Island. The danger of wishing rather than making meaningful miracles that apply to our daily lives and take into consideration the principle of complementarity extends to our culture. See Mary Catherine Bateson, "The Revenge of the Good Fairy," *Whole Earth Review* 55 (Summer 1987): 34–48.
10. As I continue to review the seventeen case records of the miracle makers whose words are included in this book, I have noted a significant cluster of characteristics that form the basis for a description of a miracologist, or someone who makes miracles. A detailed report focusing on the psychological toughness and the sleight of mind characteristics is in preparation.

    My students and colleagues have also noted that these seventeen cases reveal that each miracle maker was also a "sensuist" in that they all rejoiced in touching, holding, smelling, tasting, hearing, and seeing their world (sensualists, in contrast, are concerned only with sexual feelings). One of the most beautifully poetic and scientifically accurate books regarding the senses is Diane Ackerman's *A Natural History of the Senses* (New York: Random House, 1990).
11. O'Regan, "Healing, Remission, and Miracle Cures," 9.
12. This, and all of the quotes from patients and healthcare workers who have been a part of miracles, are drawn from my seventeen case records mentioned earlier.

13. Richard Dienstbier, "Arousal and Physiological Toughness: Implications for Mental and Physical Health," *Psychological Review* 96, no. 1 (1989): 84–100.

14. Quoted in Charles Wallis, *The Treasure Chest* (San Francisco: Harper & Row, 1983), 118.

15. William Bucke, "From Self to Cosmic Consciousness," in *The Highest State of Consciousness*, ed. J. White (Garden City, NY: Doubleday, 1972).

16. Abraham Maslow, *The Farther Reaches of Human Nature* (New York: Viking, 1971).

17. Roger Walsh, "The Psychologies of East and West: Contrasting Views of the Human Condition and Potential," in *Beyond Health and Normality*, ed. Roger Walsh and Deane Shapiro (New York: Van Nostrand Reinhold, 1983), 57.

18. Quoted in Robert Byrne, *The Third—And Possibly the Best—637 Best Things Anybody Ever Said* (New York: Antheneum, 1986), 43.

19. Bernard Siskin and Jerome Staller, *What Are the Chances?* (New York: Crown Publishers, 1989), 61.

20. M. L. von Franz, *On Divination and Synchronicity* (Toronto: Inner City Books, 1980).

21. Arnold Mindel, "Synchronicity, An Investigation of the Unitary Background Patterning Synchronous Phenomena," *Dissertation Abstracts International* 37, no. 2 (1976).

22. Werner Heisenberg, *Physics and Beyond* (New York: Harper & Row, 1971).

23. Quoted in F. David Peat, *Synchronicity. The Bridge Between Matter and Mind* (New York: Bantam Books, 1988), 28.

24. M. Scott Peck, *The Road Less Traveled* (New York: Simon & Schuster, 1976), 16.

25. Quoted in Charles Wallis, *The Treasure Chest* (San Francisco: Harper & Row, 1983), 187.

26. Buckminster Fuller, *Critical Path* (New York: St. Martin's, 1981), 26.

27. Quoted in Charles Wallis, *The Treasure Chest* (San Francisco: Harper & Row, 1983), 120.

28. Joseph Priestly, *Man and Time* (London: W. H. Allen, 1978), 245.

5
LOVE LAWS

The Science of Intensive Caring

> We often think that when we have completed our study of "one" we know all about "two," because "two" is "one and one." We forget that we still have to make a study of "and."
>
> —ARTHUR EDDINGTON

Love Support Systems

No matter how hard I tried, I could not lift my chest. The respirator was breathing for me, but something was wrong. "This is it," I thought. "I'm dying again. Just like Patsy's balloon, my lungs just will not fill with air."

I was on a life-support system and connected to several tubes, yet I felt the panic of being totally unsupported and disconnected from everything. With the tube taped to my cheek to hold it in place down my throat, I could not move my head. I struggled to cast my glance down to my chest. I saw my wife's head resting there. I felt a warmth spread through me, and I began to cry.

My sobbing awakened my wife. She had fallen asleep with her head on my chest and had slept there through the night. "Are you all right?" she asked in a sleepy voice.

"Thanks to you I am," I wrote quickly on my notepad.

"Oh, my God," she answered. "I'll bet my head was heavy on your chest. Could you breathe okay?"

I wrote, "I couldn't breathe without you."

More than tubes and electronic monitors, my wife, my family, and my friends were my real life-support system. My connection with them kept me connected to something more powerful than my illness. Their love became a force that carried me through the worst times of my life. Love created a source of energy that was so real that many of the medical people who cared for me reported actually seeing and feeling that energy and its powerful impact on my survival.

Psychologist Carl Jung wrote, "The meeting of two personalities is like the contact of two chemical substances; if there is any reaction, both are transformed."[1] In quantum physics terms, love is the force that changes us from the "particle" state of our individual experience of life to the "wave" or energy side of our living. The principle of complementarity teaches that we are both particle and wave, and I suggest that love is the name we give to the transformational force that moves us from being separate "stuff" to being connected energy. Love is the force that helps us to dance between the freedom of our "particlehood," or individual personhood, and the joy of our "wavehood," or our ability—literally—to join forces with other people.

A Science of Loving

My family's extraordinary loving stabilized my spirit (the "wave," or energy, aspect of my existence) as surely as the high-tech machines were busy stabilizing my physical body (the "particle," or matter, aspect of my existence). I would not have survived without both of these remarkable factors, and I suggest that new science provides six specific findings that not only explain the workings of the human body, the planets, and the stars, but also clarify the wonders of the power of love.

In previous chapters we have explored four basic principles of new science as they relate to miracles. The principles of nonlocality, complementarity, observer participancy, and uncertainty are four of the ten sacred secrets of science outlined in chapter 1.

In this chapter, I will introduce the remaining six secrets of science that, coincidentally, also explain the nature of loving. In chapters 6 through 11 of this book, we will explore in detail each of these six secrets as they relate to the miraculous potency of love as a healing force. Retracing the steps of my own journey from the dreadful day of my diagnosis of death to the joyful tears of celebration of my cure, I will document how loving is a key characteristic of miracle making and how it is the ultimate place where what science knows and what religion believes merge into the glory of the healing spirit.

The "Third Thing" and the "Between"

Plato wrote, "Two things alone cannot be satisfactorily united without a third; for there must be some bond between them drawing them together."[2] The "third thing" to which Plato refers is the "and" in the "one and one" equation in Eddington's quote at the beginning of this chapter. There is never just a lover and the beloved. There has to be a third thing, a miracle, that catalyzes a loving union.

Author Martin Buber refers to this third thing as the "between," or the binding force that bonds what he called the "I and the Thou" into a singular "I-Thou."[3] *Without the I-Thou union, miracle making is impossible,* because this union is the manifestation of the loving kindness shown by all miracle makers. This union, this third thing, is nonlocal loving (everywhere with everyone at all times). It is demonstrated as a deep caring for all of humanity above and beyond the narrow definition of one "self" desiring to be with another "self."

Miracle makers are well aware of the bonding power of the third thing, or the between. I recall a woman whose room was down the hall from mine on the bone marrow transplant unit. She was terribly thin, and always appeared pensive. Even when she looked directly at you, she seemed just barely to be with you. She seemed to be inviting you to go with her to another place where she was spending most of her healing time. When she walked the halls with her Christmas tree IV, she often became a part of Patsy's parade.

"My daughter's love for me and mine for her is so real that I can feel it," said this woman who so seldom smiled but always sent a message of hope. "It's like we are both plugged in to some universal energy source [nonlocality] and sharing its power. If she is in the room when I get my chemotherapy, the chemicals seem to lose their burning power. Our love power overwhelms it. Even when she is not with me, she can send her love and I can receive it. It is a thing we create between us. It's like love gravity. It's powerful, it's everywhere, it's real, and no one can defy or deny it."

The Gravity of Love

In my own case, this third thing (or in psychophysics terms, "the gravity field of the love force") was so strong that doctors and nurses actually saw it and felt it. The always-smiling nurse Betsy described one late-night encounter when the third thing appeared right before her eyes.

"You could see it," said Betsy. "Every time Dr. Pearsall and his wife were near each other, we all gravitated toward the bed. We felt the force pulling us. If you looked, you could actually see a glow between them and feel the pull. It was just like when you head straight down on a roller coaster and feel the pull."

Karen, another of my nurses, always seemed to be looking for something. Everyone seemed to count on her to find anything that was lost. Patients' files, doctors' orders, medicines, keys, or instruments were instantly found by Karen's radar. Karen said, "I think I have a homing device in my uterus or somewhere. I can beam in on things and find them. I can feel where they have hidden themselves."

"I could feel the love between Dr. Pearsall and his family," said Karen. "I felt it the way I do when I find something that has been lost. I sense a warmth and I am drawn to it. I saw something like a light between them and it pulled me there."

One doctor, whom we came to call Dr. Death Vader, was himself stunned by the power of the third thing. Dr. Death Vader was forever the cynic and skeptic. He had told me that there was no doubt I would die within days and that I should "not get my hopes up." When he said that, I always wondered where he would like me to put my hopes, if not "up."

"Okay," said Dr. Vader reluctantly and with embarrassment. "I saw a light between them, too. I felt something like an electricity. I am sure it was static electricity or maybe some type of electrochemical reaction from all the medicines and the machines."

A nurse named Beverly referred to the light that Dr. Vader saw as the "healing halo." She said, "I've seen that healing halo many times in intensive care. It looks just like the halo over the head of angels." Is it a meaningful coincidence that the painters of some of our most beautiful works of sacred art chose to use the effect of halos and emanating light to symbolize sanctity, enlightenment, conversion, and infusion with the Holy Spirit? Is this light that is so universally reported and depicted a manifestation of the fifth energy, the X-energy of the spirit that has its source in our loving?

Freedom from Particle Prison

As we lead our daily lives, we typically see ourselves as "particles" moving through space. We bump into one another and sometimes crash into one another, but we often ignore or don't believe in our "wave," or energy, side except perhaps at moments of transition, crisis, and great joy in our lives.

At particularly energized times such as birthing, dying, hurting, and healing, we may experience a "noetic explosion" in which we suddenly see our world on an energy or wave level. We are awed and often find ourselves without words to describe our feelings. These are the times when the making of miracles is possible: the times when we leap from particle to wave, from the experience of our personhood to the realization of our nonlocality.

Psychologist Dana Zohar writes, "In a quantum psychology, there are not isolated persons. Individuals do exist, do have an identity, a meaning, and a purpose, but, like particles, each of them is a brief manifestation of a particularity."[4] Medicine traditionally has viewed patients as particles and disease as a disarray of particles, but has ignored the fact that patients and disease are also forms of energy.

As described in chapter 1, the principle of complementarity tells us that we are both particle and wave, and the uncertainty principle reminds us that we become less and less certain about our wave side if we are consumed by our focus on our particle side. The more we focus on "me" (our particle side), therefore, the less we can understand and benefit from the power of "us" (our wave side). We are not just "love lumps" that "fall" in and out of love by bumping into other "love lumps."

Author François de La Rochefoucauld wrote, "Lovers never get tired of each other, because they are forever talking about themselves."[5] He meant that when we become aware of our energy or wave side, we acknowledge our oneness with another person. When we talk about someone we love, we are always really talking about "us" and not "me" or "them."

When we throw a "lump" into a pond, it creates waves or "energy jumps." When we love, our wave side is merging with the energy ripple of someone else. Like two stones thrown into a clear pond, our ripples overlap. The power generated at the juncture of overlap of our energy ripples provides the fuel for miracles.

The joy of miracles, as in all of life, is confirmed through our relationships more than through the "stuff" of our accomplishments. I rediscover the beauty of the island of Maui every time someone we love comes to visit. Sharing their joy in this paradise reawakens our own awareness of the miracle of this magical place where volcanoes, wind, rain, ocean, sun, and tropical plants combine into something far more than any one of these natural features could produce alone.

Loving the Walls Down

Plato wrote, "There is no greater or keener pleasure than that of bodily love—and none which is more irrational."[6] Bodily love is particle juxtapositioning. It is the feeling of friction between two individuals who have come into physical contact. In terms of the laws of new science, true loving is a merging of waves of energy that creates—like the fallout from a nuclear explosion—a third thing, or a love force, that radiates everywhere and "positively contaminates" everyone exposed to it. Like ripples of water merging to become more powerful waves, the "fallout" from our noetic explosions is love.

Love is two people celebrating the fact of their nonlocality. Love is evidence of action at a distance and the transcendence of time and space. Love is not limited by partitions between patients in hospitals, plastic sterile bubbles protecting patients from germs, or walls between two sides of the same country. The crumbling of the wall between West and East Germany was accomplished as much by the energy of the human spirit and by the irresistible longings of people wanting to be with people as by political negotiation.

If you are in love, you can feel the presence of your lover right now by simply paying attention to your lover's imprint on your spirit. If any more proof of nonlocality were needed, the "third thing" or the "between" is that proof. Time or distance cannot separate lovers.

Philosopher Pir Vilayatkhan writes, "The assumption of being an individual is our greatest limitation."7 Unfortunately, like much of our living, loving has been explained on an "old science" bias. This bias has limited us to a physical, frictional, particle, individualistic view of love, and out of this view has come divorce, infidelity, and spouse abuse. If we limit ourselves to a particle point of view, then we only bump into each other rather than merge.

One MM said, "I'm sick of bump and rub love. We run into each other, rub for a little while to create some friction and heat, get too hot, burn out, and cool off, and then split. I'm looking for some quantum loving where there is more lasting energy and more merging."8

An Old Science of Loving

The famous *cogito ergo sum* or "I think, therefore I am" phrase of Descartes stresses the knowing of an "I" that is a local and ultimately lonely self. There can be no intimate connection between two people "meeting I to I." This local thinking is echoed by modern psychology, which often follows the notion of "I do my thing and you do your thing. You are you and I am I."9 This philosophy has left us a lonely legacy of selfishness, narcissism, and a continuing difficulty in maintaining loving relationships.

Many of the diseases of civilization such as cancer, heart disease, stroke, and diabetes are also partly disorders of loving. All healthy cells in our body must sacrifice themselves for the good of the whole body system by controlling their growth and altering their function so that a system rather than a selfish set of destructive cells is the end result. In a sense, the cancer cell has failed to "love," and develops a chemistry of narcissism. It functions as if it were alone outside the unity of the body system. It becomes malignant and spreads wildly and destructively throughout the body because it uses rather than merges with the system from which it sprung.

We often look for lovers to meet our sexual and romantic appetite rather than to merge with us meaningfully and spiritually in the nonlocal sense described in this book. Like cells behaving selfishly, we keep spreading out but never merge. Some individuals attempt to find love by littering their lives with broken relationships, *searching* for the right person instead of trying to *be* the right person.

"I don't know about having affairs," said one of the male MMs who had been in and out of several of what he called "liaisons" or brief sexual affairs. Even on the hospital unit, he would be, in his words, "cruising and casing the halls rather than exercising." Following his illness, however, he said "Affairs are hot as hell, and you can't beat the excitement. But I can tell you now that I don't think anyone in any of my affairs would be cleaning up my vomit after chemotherapy or sensing just exactly when I need my pain medicine like my wife does. What you really need is real love that goes beyond just two people. You create something between the two of you that is more than the two of you and it keeps the two of you alive."

Sir Isaac Newton's physics, like Descartes's philosophy, is a science of isolation. He taught that matter is made up of particles that, like the planets, move separately through their individual and predictable orbits governed by purely mechanical laws of gravity and linear time. "Stuff" might collide on occasion, but these collisions cause only a mild change of direction and speed. The stuff that collides is not altered or, as Jung suggested, "transformed."

We are conditioned to see love as a series of mechanical adjustments made as a result of collision with our lover. Too few of us understand nonlocal loving and realize that changes in our basic nature occur when we collide with another particle person. We find ourselves in Newtonian space when we use love postures of "getting next to," or "on top of" each other. We try to "get inside" each other or allow someone to get inside us, but this is a penetration of position and posture, not a merging of energy.

As a counterreaction to Cartesian-Newtonian loving, artists and musicians have tended to romanticize love in their songs, paintings, and poems. They imply that, if there is any "self-altering" in our loving, it is a mystical, rare, overwhelming, and even debilitating love sickness. Such loving is almost always temporary. I recently overheard two teenagers talking. The girl said, "You told me you loved me once." The young love mechanic answered, "That was the once." This is an example of the transitional love collisions that have become all too common.

Toward Quantum Love

As newborn babies, we craved closeness with our mothers. In the absence of that closeness, we feel fear and helplessness. As adults, we continue to long for closeness but also fear that we will lose our identity if we become "too close" or "too much a part" of someone else. Like the gambling I described in chapter 4 as a process necessary for giving meaning to the coincidences of our lives, making the miracle of quantum, or a true merging, love requires that we gamble in our loving. We must take the risk that a love will not work out or that some crisis will disrupt the physical manifestations of that love, yet know that the process of a merging, energetic loving is worth the pain.

Parents know about the gamble of quantum love. They know that there is always pain, worry, and loss in their loving of their children. One of the mothers of a teenage bone marrow transplant patient said, "There have been so many times when I have almost regretted having her. I mean, I love her so, and watching her suffer like this causes me to hurt so deeply with her that I almost wish that I would have never had children. But then I know it is because she is and always will be a part of me that I feel such pain, and I remember the loving we share and how there really isn't anything to life other than the people who are a part of you forever. Relationships are the only thing that really count."

Like all miracle makers, this loving mother took the gamble of loving self and other as one and making a third thing out of the composite. Quantum (wave) love, the joining of spiritual energy with all of its joy and pain, is a celebration of "us." Whereas narcissistic (particle) love is often characterized by the "just you and me against the world" approach, quantum love is the "us with the world" approach.

Following a recent lecture, an old Jewish gentleman approached me. He said, "Do you know the story of Jehovah and Abraham's argument?" I confessed I did not, and he said, "Then let me tell you about it, because it makes your point about needing an "us" to make a miracle."

In a strong Yiddish accent, the old man began his story, and everyone around listened in. "You see, Jehovah and Abraham were arguing about who is most responsible for our wonderful world. Jehovah reminds Abraham that Abraham would not exist if it were not for him, Jehovah. Abraham says he knows he owes his very existence to Jehovah, and adds, 'But also, you would not be known if it were not for me.' You see, it always takes an 'us,' " finished the old man. [10] As the MM who had many liaisons told me, "What good would this whole miracle of my getting better be if I couldn't share it? It would be like having the most fantastic secret in the world that you could never share with anyone." *Loving is the sharing of miracles.* Every miracle I experienced or have studied had one characteristic in common: It resulted from and enhanced the third thing.

Miracles and the New Science of Loving

The love described by the laws of new science is a love free of striving for here-and-now satisfaction. It also is free of the linear, cause-and-effect rule of "If you love me, then I will love you."

Miracle love happens when a miracle maker *makes a choice* to actively create love by seeing love everywhere, not waiting to "fall into it" or for it to "happen to" him or her. Miracle makers have "the look" or vision of loving and their loving point of view causes love to happen (observer participantcy).

Miracle love follows the principle of complementarity in that it embraces all that a lover is and all aspects of loving. Anger, impatience, and conflict are complementary to the tolerance, acceptance, and patience of quantum loving. Quantum loving is not a loving of failed expectation or rejection when the beloved falls short of perfection. Instead, quantum love looks at loving from both of its complementary sides, including all of the challenges to loving. It endures in sickness and in health, for richer and for poorer, but it is not broken by physical death. Miracle love is infinite (principle of nonlocality).

Miracle love follows the principle of uncertainty in acknowledging that the more we think we know about those we love, the more there is about them that we do not yet know. I have noticed that one of the best predictors of Cartesian-Newtonian lovers about to fall out of their local loving is when they start believing that they know everything about their lover that there is to know. "I know him better than I know myself" is a statement that may signal that there is much more about your lover that is available for discovery, if you are willing to take the gamble of continuing to look for it. It is a gamble to keep learning about your lover because you will learn the bad with the good. The test is of *you*, not your lover, and you pass the test if you can achieve a quantum loving of your whole lover, not his or her selected characteristics.

In the previous chapter, I outlined six characteristics of a miracle maker. The seventh characteristic of miracle makers is their capacity for loving kindness and their ability to mobilize the third thing—the force of love—for healing, happiness, and hope.

Miracle makers like Patsy make powerful, lasting connections with those around them. They are "magnetic," drawing people and healing energy toward them as much as they give off this same energy. The remainder of this chapter will introduce six science principles that helped Patsy, the MMs, and me make our miracles. They are also the secrets of making quantum love. When these six principles, outlined below, are combined with the four general theories of nonlocality, observer participantcy, complementarity, and uncertainty, already discussed, we uncover the ten sacred secrets of science or of miracle making.

Science Principle Number One: Oneness

In the quantum world—the world of the very, very small going very, very fast—there is no such thing as "isolation." The central quantum principle is that everything and everyone is one. While individuality does exist, it has no meaning without the context of connection.

One of the major figures in new science is Max Planck, who originated many of the theories of quantum mechanics. Planck suggested that the universe is not continuous or made up of parts linked one to the other by time and through space. He showed that "quantum," or energy and particle "spurts," exist, and that "quantum leaps" that transcend space and time were possible in a "multiple track" universe of many realities. He wrote that ultimately everything in the universe is "one."[11] Max Planck knew that the universe is not a vacuum of emptiness. It is everything going on all at once and together. When physicist Erwin Schrödinger coined the term "One Mind,"[12] he meant that all of the laws of physics point to one incontrovertible fact: We are all One. You will see in chapter 6 that a key step in making miracles is to perceive our world as one mind with billions of individual "brain" contributors to the whole rather than a world populated by 5 billion individual and local brains. We share a "mind" and consciousness with the objects around us, particularly with animals and plants. Consider, for example, the work of Charles Darwin as outlined in *The Expression of the Emotions in Man and Animals.* Darwin wrote of the Indian elephant, "When over-powered and made fast, his grief was most affecting; his violence sank to utter prostration, and he lay on the ground, uttering choking cries, with tears trickling down his cheeks."[13] Can you feel a oneness with the experience of this wonderful animal?

Author and poet Heathcote Williams wrote of our oneness and shared spirit with whales and elephants.[14] Williams explores the meaning of the fact that elephants cry, conduct autopsies on their dead, have processional funerals, and even draw on the walls of their cages. We, the elephants, and everything are drawn together in oneness. The motto of the miracle maker is All are one; in one are all!

Science Principle Number Two: Realms of Reality

Quantum physics gave birth to what is referred to as the "Many Worlds" theory. Philosopher and scientist John White has identified what he calls seven levels of spirituality.[15] These seven realms are the *physical* laws of mass and energy, *biological* (the laws of basic life processes), *psychological* (the laws of the developing self), *sociological* (the laws of interaction between all of us), *ecological* (the interactive laws of scientist and futurist Buckminster Fuller's "spaceship earth"), *cosmological* (the laws of the flow of energy between the stars and planets of the universe), and *theological* (the laws of our interaction with God). Too often, scientists and theologians alike suffer from "domain lock" and fail to draw from the lessons of all seven sources of our spiritual development. In chapter 7, I will focus on five of the many realms of reality that are particularly relevant to the making of miracles.[16]

New Science principles prove (and religion believes) that the self exists in an infinite number of worlds, not just the here-and-now, see-and-touch world. We have come to rely on what we can see because two-thirds of all nerve fibers entering the human central nervous system come from the eyes.[17] We have come to rely on our sense of touch because the dendrites or neurological fibers that react to external stimulation operate by reflex and without thought. But these two senses bring us only two of the available worlds of reality. Our brain contains a *potential* number of interconnections greater than the number of atoms in the entire universe![18] We learn to make miracles by taking conscious control of our brains and by making our own connections with other realities through our chosen observations.

Psychologists refer to four states of consciousness. They describe waking, sleeping, dreaming, and what is sometimes called the fourth or "uncommon consciousness." This is a state of altered awareness often associated with miracles, profound insight, distant viewing, forecasting the future, and psychic phenomenon (psi). Thus it appears that there may be as many different realities as there are ways to see them.

Author Diane Ackerman writes, "One of the greatest sensuists [someone who rejoices in sensory experiences] of all time . . . was a handicapped woman with several senses gone."[19] Ackerman is describing Helen Keller, who, in spite of being blind, deaf, and mute, could hold a radio in her hands and feel the difference between the violins and the trumpets and "feel" the stories of Mark Twain as he described the wonders of the Mississippi River. Helen Keller was a miracle maker because she could travel through many realms of reality and free herself from the trap of seeing just with the eyes and hearing only with the ears. You will be able to learn this same skill by following some of the suggestions in chapter 7.

Science Principle Number Three: Simultaneity

Two of the most remarkable findings from new physics are that time is relative and that simultaneity is possible. It is a scientific fact that it is only on one of the levels of reality—that of the see-and-touch world—that time seems to be linear and flowing. In other realities, things happen all at once, and the present and future can determine the past.

Historian W. Warren Wagar studies the present by casting his glance back from the future.[20] From the view of a twenty-second-century historian, Wagar looks back on the future to examine giant Japanese-American megacorporations, a global economy, the dangers of sharing a world without sharing a common faith in goodness, and even the near-fatal epidemic of continual animal eating that nearly wiped out the civilizations of the "old days" of the twenty-first century. By refusing to follow historians' typical orientation of looking back at time from the present, Wagar was able to leap forward to look backward. By choosing this form of observation, he was able, in effect, to create a past. In chapter 8, you will see how miracle makers have this same capacity for time travel in their own perceptions.

The concept of simultaneity and our freedom from the limits of distance and time are collectively referred to as Bell's Theorem. This theorem suggests that there is a synchronized dance across time and space that defies our cause-and-effect orientation to daily living.[21] In physics, any photon (a quantum or particle of light energy) always has a partner somewhere in the universe. If the direction of the photon's spin is changed, it will be joined in that change by its partner *no matter where the partner may be*. This change is instantaneous! Chapter 9 will describe the miracle-making power of understanding this remarkable timelessness that governs our human spirits.

Science Principle Number Four: Forceful Fields

The idea that invisible fields directly affect our lives is now accepted by all of science. Gravitational fields and electromagnetic fields affect everything from the ebb and flow of the tides to the flow of energy through electric power lines. Recent research indicates that the invisible electromagnetic fields from high tension wires and even extreme low frequency (ELF) fields may be implicated as a cause of certain forms of cancer. In this case, some invisible field has seriously altered the cells in the human body. You are not able to "see" these force fields, but their effect is immediate, consistent, and powerful.

In chapter 9, you will read about the work of Rupert Sheldrake, a young plant physiologist from England. Sheldrake suggests that we are much more than biochemical, molecular systems. He proposes that we are as we are because we are surrounded by resonating fields to which we can tune in. He carefully reviews a mass of evidence in support of the fact that animals have passed on their *learned* behaviors to their offspring through what he calls "morphogenesis" or fields of influence above and beyond the cell and the gene. He cites one classic case (also recounted by Charles Darwin) of how a mastiff dog who was mistreated by a butcher developed a dislike for all butchers and butcher shops, and how this "butcher-phobia" carried through several generations of the mastiff's line.[22]

I suggest that many forms of illness are times when our morphogenetic fields, or energy fields, are reorganizing and readjusting. We are getting back into the shape that our fields direct us to be in. As you will read in chapter 9, even the life-threatening disease of cancer involves the influence of these reorganizing fields. Miracle makers can tune into these forces to maximize healing.

Science Principle Number Five: Divine Dynamics

The First Law of Thermodynamics is that energy cannot be created or destroyed. If you hang a bowling ball from a rope, suspend the rope from an almost frictionless pulley on the ceiling, pull the ball back to your nose and let the ball swing free, the ball will move out like a pendulum and back to exactly the same point in front of your nose from which it was released. (As they warn on television shows, however, I would not suggest that you try this experiment at home. If you make just a small miscalculation by hanging the ball with too much friction, pushing the ball instead of just letting it go, or flinch and move toward the ball just slightly, your career in the study of thermodynamics could be over!)

The First Law of Thermodynamics holds up very well in almost all experiments and applies very well to our daily lives. While we might be going through constant change, there is only all the energy and matter that there ever was after the Big Bang. In contrast, the Second Law of Thermodynamics, which suggests that entropy, or disorganization, is always increasing toward ultimate destruction in the form of cosmic burnout, does not apply well to our daily lives.

Although inanimate objects do seem to move toward a state of maximum disorder (entropy), living systems move through disorder as a path toward more order. As one of the MMs said, "We have to get messed up so we can get in better order." Entropy (moving through disorganization and flux) is a necessary process of healthy living because it is a form of shuffling the cards for a new and better hand to play in the game of life.

In chapter 10, you will learn that the energy of our living may throw things into disarray, but that a new order always emerges. As physicist Harold Morowitz writes, "The flow of energy through a system acts to organize (not disorganize) that system."[23] Miracle makers welcome disarray as a challenge, a form of divine dynamics required to make more miracles rather than as a sign that their world is falling apart.

Science Principle Number Six: Love and Order

Growing out of the study of patterns of entropy is one of the newest fields of "new science" referred to as chaos theory. This theory suggests that the apparently random, unpredictable nature of our living, loving, crises, and healing masks an ultimate, awesome, and magnificently beautiful order. "Divine dynamics" suggests that the disarray in our living and loving is a symptom that we are moving toward a higher order. The law of chaotic order suggests that chaos—the actual process of disorder—is healthy in and of itself. The universe is not a beautiful balance; it is a chaotic miracle.

Maintaining our faith in this ultimate order beneath the chaos and learning to appreciate—even celebrate—the state of chaos itself is a major component of miracle making. This faith need not be a blind faith, for as you have seen, there are many new science principles to help us understand the sudden breakthroughs of order that come in the form of meaningful coincidences. Scientist Douglas Hofstadter writes, "It turns out that an eerie type of chaos can lurk just behind a facade of order—and yet, deep inside the chaos lurks an even eerier type of order."[24]

During one of my chemotherapy treatments, I was reading

James Gleick's book *Chaos*, which describes the evolution of this new science. I was just beginning to read chapter 1 when, as often happened when the chemicals began to burn my veins, my arm began to tremor. I dropped the book. My wife picked it up and handed it to me. I opened it at random. The first passage I read was a quote from psychiatrist Arnold Mandell: "Is it possible that mathematical pathology, i.e. chaos, is health?"[25] In chapter 11, I will explore the paradox that we do not really find meaning in chaos—chaos *is* the meaning of our life! Miracle makers find a majestic beauty in the whirls, twirls, and scattered flurries of our chaotic life.

I was undergoing the strongest form of chemotherapy available for the cancer that was causing chaos in my body, but the chemotherapy itself was causing *more* chaos. I was being given medicine that reestablished equilibrium by getting into my system and stirring things up to a healthier new order in which the sick cells were crowded out by a new army of healthy cells. I remembered a statement by the same psychiatrist whose words I had stumbled on earlier. Describing the necessity of chaos, Dr. Mandell said, "When you reach an equilibrium in biology, you're dead."[26] Through the sixth secret of science, we learn that chaos is life.

The Four Questions of Crisis

When our lives seem to be beyond any meaning and when chaos overwhelms us, we ask four basic questions that always occur to us at times of despair. I asked these same four questions every day as I went from life to death and back again: "Why me? Why now? Now what? and So what?" As I take you with me through the miracles in the rest of this book, we will explore how these sacred secrets of science enrich our living and loving and even provide solutions to these four "questions of crisis." I hope you will discover, as I did, that it is when we are most deeply immersed in despair that we are the most poised on the threshold of miracles.

NOTES

1. Carl Jung, *Analytical Psychology: Its Theory and Practice: The Tavistock Lectures* (New York: Random House, 1968).

2. Plato, *The Collected Dialogues*, ed. Edith Hamilton and Huntington Cairns, Bollingen Series no. LXXI (New York: Pantheon Books, 1961).

3. Martin Buber, *I and Thou* (Edinburgh, UK: T. & T. Clark, 1937).

4. Danah Zohar, *The Quantum Self. Human Nature and Consciousness Defined by the New Physics* (New York: William Morrow, 1990), 169.

5. Quoted in William Safire and Leonard Safire, *Words of Wisdom* (New York: Simon & Schuster, 1989), 120.

6. Plato, *The Republic*, Book II.

7. Quoted in Danah Zohar, *The Quantum Self*, 107.

8. In my study of the seventeen miracle makers, I discovered their concept of "quantum loving." An entire theory of intimacy and interpersonal relationships may be developed from the metaphor of quantum science, and I am preparing a report on a "new science of loving" and the relationship between "quantum loving" and lasting relationships.

9. This approach to interpersonal relationships was made popular by the Gestalt psychology movement. The leader of this movement was Frederick Perls. See his *Gestalt Therapy Verbatim* (New York: Bantam Books, 1969).

10. This Hebrew legend is recounted in physicist John Archibald Wheeler's article "Beyond the Black Hole." He uses the story as an example of observer participantcy and the fact of our ultimate oneness. The article is printed in Harry Wolf, ed. *Some Strangeness in the Proportion* (Reading, MA: Addison-Wesley, 1980).

11. For a description of Max Planck's views of the multiple levels and wholeness of the universe, see F. F. Hoveyda, "The Image of Science in Our Society," *Biosciences Communications III* no. 3 (1977): 5–51.

12. Erwin Schrödinger, *What is Life? and Mind and Matter* (London: Cambridge University Press, 1969), 145.

13. Quoted in *Whole Earth Review* no. 67 (Summer 1990): 42.

14. A powerful case for our oneness with everything, particularly animals, is made in Heathcote Williams, *Sacred Elephant* (New York: Crown Publishers, 1989). See also his earlier book, *Whale Nation*.

15. John White, *The Meeting of Science and Spirit: The Next Dynamic Stage of Human Evolution and How We Will Attain It* (New York: Paragon House, 1990), 239.

16. Different domains of reality are described in the work by Lawrence LeShan and Henry Margenau, *Einstein's Space and Van Gogh's Sky: Physical Reality and Beyond* (New York: Macmillan, 1982).

17. R. Gerard, "Units and Concepts of Biology," *Science* 125 (1957): 429–433.

18. Robert Ornstein, *Psychology: The Study of Human Experience* (New York: Harcourt Brace Jovanovich, 1988), 133.

19. Diane Ackerman, *A Natural History of the Senses* (New York: Random House, 1990), xviii.
20. W. Warren Wagar, *A Short History of the Future* (Chicago: University of Chicago Press, 1989).
21. An example of the research on the startling Bell's Theorem and our capacity to experience simultaneity and a freedom from linear time is in R. I. Pfleegor and L. Mandel, "Interference of Independent Photon Beams," *Physical Review* 159, no. 5 (1967).
22. Rupert Sheldrake, *The Presence of the Past* (New York: Random House, 1988).
23. Harold Morowitz, *Energy Flow in Biology* (Woodridge, CT: Ox Bow Press, 1979).
24. Douglas R. Hofstadter, *Metamagical Themas* (New York: Basic Books, 1985), 233.
25. James Gleick, *Chaos: Making a New Science* (New York: Penguin Books, 1987), 298. This book provides a remarkable discussion of chaos theory.
26. Arnold J. Mandell, "From Molecular Biological Simplification to More Realistic Central Nervous System Dynamics: An Opinion," in *Psychiatry: Psychobiological Foundations of Clinical Psychiatry,* vol. 3, no. 2, ed. J. O. Cavenar *et al.* (Philadelphia: Lippincott, 1985).

6

LIFE'S MOST IMPORTANT CHOICE

My Will or Thy Will Be Done

No matter where you go, there you are.
—BUMPER STICKER

One Hundred Monkeys Can't Be Wrong

In the late 1970s, the Japanese government maintained small colonies of Philippine macaques (monkeys) in order to study their habits. A young female monkey named Ima discovered how to clean sand and dirt from sweet potatoes by dunking and washing them in a stream. She taught this skill one at a time to several other monkeys. Suddenly, after 100 monkeys learned Ima's potato-washing technique, a *quantum leap* in this monkey skill took place and *every monkey* in the entire colony was *instantly* able to wash potatoes!

Respected biologist Lyle Watson described the suddenness of this monkey "oneness" and the "hundredth monkey phenomenon" as follows: "The number of potato washers was 99 and at 11 o'clock on Tuesday morning, one further convert was added to the fold in the usual way [learning from Ima]. The addition of the hundredth monkey apparently carried the number across some critical mass, because by that evening almost everyone in the colony was doing it."[1] Even more surprising is the fact that the potato-washing skill, according to Watson, "seems to have jumped natural barriers [time and space] and to have appeared spontaneously in colonies on other islands and on the mainland."[2]

This chapter will illustrate how the science secret of oneness can unleash powerful healing forces that take quantum leaps across the barriers of time and space.

A Key Choice

The nature and quality of your entire life is determined by your answer to the following question: Are you an "I" or an "Us?" The idea that we are a part of everyone and everything should be the ultimate source of comfort and celebration, yet we often seem to think that our personal security rests with being a rugged and self-sufficient individualist. The Arabian proverb, "Trust in Allah, but tie your camel," reflects the idea that we should believe in the power of our oneness with God but be ever vigilant for the protection of our "real self" and those things and people that we think belong to us here and now.

Particularly in this country, built as it is on the pioneer spirit, we tend to think that our safety depends on our self-sufficiency. I promise you, however, that at times of severe crisis and at times when you need a miracle the most, the fact of your oneness with the universe will be driven home with force. You will feel the power of prayer, even if those persons praying for you are miles away. You will feel the need for the loving care of others, and you will sense, as I did, that when you are the most afraid, your inner need for a connection with others is the strongest.

Our Shared Self

Physicist Erwin Schrödinger's One Mind concept referred to in chapter 5 implies that "The localization of the personality, of the conscious mind, inside the body is only symbolic, just an aid for practical use."[3] We seem to feel that our "self" is somewhere just inside us, or as Schrödinger writes, "an inch or two behind the midpoint of the eyes." Such a view fits well with a mechanical view of living, but it ignores the fact that separateness is not possible because it violates the scientific fact of oneness.

It can be frightening to contemplate the boundlessness of a space-and-time–free universal Self that shares One Mind. When we realize that our cause-and-effect world is only one convenient way of ordering our lives and that we are united on a more profound level with all of the cosmos in an existence that is neither local (here and now) nor certain, we feel insecure and awed by the possibilities of life. It is easy to give in to the pseudosecurity of a locally housed self. But the self is not "there" or "here" in any one place. Science teaches us that the self is nonlocal and everywhere.

The Enchanted Loom

Paradoxically, the evidence for the One Mind rather than the 5 billion separate brains view is supported by the fact that we always experience our consciousness in the singular. Dr. Schrödinger writes, "Not only has none of us ever experienced more than one consciousness at the same time, but there is also no trace of circumstantial evidence that this ever happened anywhere in the world."[4]

If you reflect on your own experience of love, hate, worry, fear, or hope, you will notice that it's not an "us" that feels these emotions, but what we call an "I." This "I" is not an isolated self. It is a singular pronoun for the way we *all* experience these emotions.

Like the "enchanted loom" model of One Mind suggested by the famous neurological scientist Sir Charles Sherrington, we are forever woven and weaving together. One of the clearest signals that a readjustment in our spiritual growth is taking place should be the sense that we are becoming "unraveled" or in some way disconnected from others and the world. When we begin to feel disconnected, it is a cry from our spirit to be put back together again with everyone and everything and to be sewn back into the collective soul.

My Miracle Journey Begins

My sickness and healing began on August 8, 1988, when I noticed the slightest twitch of discomfort in the upper-middle area of my back, just between my shoulder blades. By coincidence, spiritual leaders throughout the world were placing great hope and significance on the same date when I first felt this pain, at about 8:00 P.M. Hawaiian time. The eighth day of the eighth month of the eighty-eighth year of this century was being targeted as a time for shared consciousness for the improvement of our planet, and that date of 8/8/88 at 8:00 P.M. will always be fixed in my mind. Hundreds of people had come to Haleakala volcano behind my Maui home to attempt to join their consciousness in creating peace, love, and preservation of the planet. At exactly that same time, I was to begin my own journey of miracles.

Again by coincidence, twenty-five years earlier, I had become engaged to my wife on August 8 at about 8:00 A.M. in a rose garden on the University of Michigan campus. Now, I was at a new crossroads, finally celebrating my new career as author and lecturer living half-time in the paradise of Maui, Hawaii. I was living where people came to enhance their cosmic consciousness, and my own consciousness was being challenged as never before.

I was leaving the clinic that I had founded, designed, and directed at a major hospital in Detroit. Doing this was extremely difficult. New leadership had come to the general hospital some years before, and the economic crisis in medicine was necessitating a "bottom line economics" mentality. Administrators and accountants who had never seen a patient were making decisions that would alter patient care forever. If I left, it was likely that the hospital would have to close the clinic. In order to start a new dream, I would have to end another, and the emotional pain was severe.

In my last weeks of directing the clinic, I felt a deep sense of disappointment and disconnection from my staff and the thousands of patients whom we had helped. Once in Maui, even though I was surfing, swimming, writing, lecturing, and spending time with my family, I still felt strangely disconnected and disoriented. Starting my new dream life was exciting, however, and the excitement distracted me from seeing how alienated I felt as one of the major periods of my life drew to a painful close.

I do not suggest that my feelings of disconnection directly caused the beginning of my illness, but the coincidence of the time and date, the metaphor of connecting, and the order and power (according to Kammerer's coincidence classification concepts) of the coincidental series of eights provided a hint as to what would later provide many of my miracles. It was time to find a new order and meaning in my life. It was time to form a new understanding of the purpose of my life, and it was an opportunity to reaffirm my connection with my family.

As we have discussed, meaningful coincidences are clues to miracles. I believe now, after all of my suffering, that we are better off looking for clues to miracles than for explanations when crisis threatens us. I had to learn that the crises of my life were challenges to find new meaning and unity with others rather than to search for blame, sources of my own guilt, or local and singular causes for my situation. The local path through crisis leads to selfishness, defensiveness, and doubt. The path to miracles is made by being open to our oneness even when we feel the most isolated and confused.

The End of the Beginning

The pain in my back worsened. Weeks passed as the pain became so severe that sleeping, walking, and even thinking became difficult. I took painkillers of every kind, but nothing eased my suffering. Everything in my life seemed to come to a halt as the pain burned like a knife in the middle of my back. I had just begun a new life, but now everything seemed to be in chaos. "The beginning is already ending," I thought to myself in despair.

My decision to leave the Problems of Daily Living Clinic did result in its closing. Hundreds of patients called to complain, and I felt guilty for not continuing as director. My decision also resulted in the sudden ending of a major national program, and decades of work and commitment ended without ceremony. Staff, patients, and secretaries cried, and my own secretary and friend for years was suddenly reassigned to another department even before my last workday. My associate chief, a young psychiatrist, died suddenly and unexpectedly, leaving a wife and children alone. Within days, a vibrant treatment center became a suite of empty offices.

I was sick, in pain, unable to lift folders and files to clean out my office. The closing of the clinic was literally breaking my back. The department of psychiatry presented me with a parting gift of a rare tree, but (by coincidence) its trunk was broken. I left the tree in the empty clinic and my sons helped me pack my books. Thus more than twenty years of work ended. I had expected this major program would last forever, and that when I moved on, it would continue to grow. Now, I felt that my pain was a type of punishment for abandoning one dream to pursue another.

My back pain was almost unbearable. I became hostile to my own family, withdrawn from friends and colleagues, and felt helpless and alone. One of the worst aspects of pain is its potential to draw you away from your connection with others just when you need them the most. The more local and lonely I felt, the more the pain worsened. I needed what physician Larry Dossey calls the "spiritual morphine" of feeling connected and protected by my nonlocality and oneness.

Four questions began to cycle through my mind. Each of these questions had answers that I now know can be found in the new science of our spirituality. I now call them the four questions of crisis.

Oneness and Why Me?

We all ask the "Why me?" question when things go wrong in our lives. Even during good times, we may doubt our luck and ask, "Why am I getting all this good stuff?"

We may ask a version of the "Why me?" question—Why him or her?—on behalf of our loved ones when they are hurting. We may ask why such loving, good people should suffer so. Why do innocent children and tender, giving persons have to suffer? Haven't they earned some type of insult immunity?

The oneness principle of new science holds an answer. If we all are one, there is no *me*. When we suffer, we suffer as a part of, and representative of, the whole. We are not alone, an innocent target of the random distribution of suffering. Pain and joy are universal, and all of us have and will have both. The question "Why me?" should be rephrased to "Why us?" The answer then becomes, "Because we are all changing and growing forever through an array of spiritual experiences."

When I was trapped in the bone marrow transplant unit for more than eight weeks, I envied the doctors and nurses who came and went to their homes. I envied them being able to wear regular clothes, to joke, and to lead a normal life. I kept asking over and over again, "Why am I trapped and they are free? They take their freedom so much for granted."

When I confided in one of my nurses and told her of my resentment of those persons who were not sick, she answered very briefly, "Oh, come on. It's just your turn. We all go through everything in some way some time. That's just the way it is. We're all in this with you. You're not alone."

The Analgesia of Connection

As my pain became worse, I noticed a fascinating change. I began to feel more and more connected. When my pain began and was very local and mild compared to what it would be, I felt that I was suffering separately. When the pain grew to major league caliber, my whole perspective on my place in the universe started to change because of the chaos of my suffering.

My pain seemed to be spinning me to new perspectives on my life. When my eyes were closed, I felt that I was flying through the universe and was a part of the stars. By another coincidence, I received a little booklet while I was in the hospital, and I could relate to the perspective on life presented in that pamphlet.[5] The author, Guy Ottewell, suggests that we hold a piece of popcorn in our hand to represent the earth and place a bowling ball on the ground to represent the sun. To achieve the proper scale distance, we would have to take our piece of popcorn more than one-quarter of a football field away from the bowling ball. The planet Pluto would be a pinhead held ten football fields away! This feeling of immense expansiveness, and the way in which Ottewell's perspectives made our oneness with this cosmic scale comprehensible helped me to see that, as terrible as I was feeling, I was a part of a grand system that transcended my local pain. I wanted more than ever to feel a part of the overall universe as a means of transcending the local torment of my tortured body.

My earlier cries of "Leave me alone" became "Don't leave," "Hold me," and "Join me." I became "affection assertive," almost demanding that people feel with me and share with me. I began to learn the nurse's lesson of "just going through my turn." Like a painkiller or analgesic, the more my pain, the more my sense of connection seemed to lessen my pain. The more I became connected, the more easily I could manage the painful times.

Dr. Dossey writes that when we are ill we are not, "an isolated entity who is fragmented from the world of the healthy and who is adrift in flowing time, moving slowly toward extermination."[6] When you or people you love begin to ask "Why me?" recognize the danger of this disconnection and help them learn that whatever is happening is not just happening to them alone. If there is a question to be asked, it is better put "Why us?" Tell them, "This is us suffering together. You're doing the work, but we'll help and share and feel with you as much as we can. We will never be separate from you."

Oneness and "Why Now?"

As I struggled with the "Why me?" question and began to understand how therapeutic my connection with everyone was, I still wondered "Why now?" Just when I was ready to reap the fruits of years of work and research, just when I had completed my dream home in Maui, just when I had formed and directed one of the unique treatment centers in the country, just when I had completed writing several successful books and was ready to write several other books, just when I was in demand for national television shows and lectures, I had become seriously ill. This seemed to be the worst of times for the worst of times.

When I was on the bone marrow transplant unit, I learned that every patient asked the "Why now?" question. Every one of the seventeen MMs also had asked this question. It became obvious that, if we were all asking why me and why now, it was because *everyone* suffers and experiences pain and joy some time. One of the MMs said:

> I used to stay awake at night trying to figure out why I had gotten sick now, of all times. I had just gotten married, just started my job, and was just getting started in life—and bang. I've got cancer. Then I realized something obvious. Everyone was asking the same question about why now, but they were all at different stages of their life. Why just when I had a baby, why just when I retired, why just when I fell in love. The times changed, but the same question remained. There is no right time for a bad time. If you could pick a time for a crisis, when would you pick?

Imagine how we would live and feel if we were placed in charge of assigning the times for the crises in everyones' lives. Fortunately, chaos shuffles the cards for us so that we don't have to cope with the trauma of choosing the nature or the timing of our crises. We don't and can't tell the universe what to do; we can only be a part of the doing.

If we are all connected over time and space, all part of a unified One, then the concept of "now" becomes irrelevant. Whenever anything "happens" to us, it has to be the perfect time for it to happen just because it is happening. As Patsy's principle suggests, "It's just the way it is." We are thinking too locally when we think that our own personal version of time is the "right" time and that we can judge when things should and should not take place. Everything is happening all of the time to everyone. Chaos is always dealing out the cards.

Imagine that you could write the script of the rest of your life and create your own personal epoch. Suppose you could write any script you like so long as you include three terrible times of life and three very good times of life scattered among an average, linear, local life. Exactly when would you schedule in your crisis time? Would you schedule crises around the time of courtship, marriage, child rearing, career development, or perhaps just at the time you retire? When is a good time for bad things? The answer is obvious. It is pure egocentrism to think that we could come up with a better time frame for our crises and joy than the universe does.

With the humor and insight typical of miracle makers, one MM said, "I sure am glad I'm not in charge of life and living. I'll be damned if I would be able to tell when to put somebody through the hell I'm going through now. I have enough trouble managing my pizzeria. I don't think I'd want to have the universe franchise."

Little Patsy illustrated this same kind of acceptance when one of her childhood friends came to visit. "I wouldn't want to be sick now when I'm just a little kid," said the young girl. "I want to play and stuff. The old people here should be the sick ones, not you. You're a kid."

"It's just how it is," answered Patsy. "It's just the way. Everybody gets everything all of the time and any time. You don't run it, you just do it."

Just as we are one, so our life is one. It is not divided into predictable, "correct" steps to ultimate death. None of us will lead a perfect, trouble- and illness-free life, love and work, and then die quietly in our sleep at age 100 as a fulfilled individual. As you will read later, to wish for such a life may actually be dangerous to your own well-being and ultimate happiness.

As I lay alone in the darkness of my hospital room every night for almost eighty nights, the oneness of my life became clearer. I realized that now was the perfect time to be sick. Now was the time for readjustment. Once I accepted Patsy's "the way it is," much of the pressure to "get well fast" or "get past this terrible time and move on" was relieved. Once I was free of trying to live quickly through this time, I could become immersed in the process of trying to make a miracle from it. I became able to grasp the moment rather than try to outrun my illness. By doing so I could benefit from the loving, praying, and healing offered from everyone who cared for and was one with me.

As difficult as it is to accept, crises are meaningful coincidences in our life as much as are the unexpected breakthroughs of joy. Meaningful miracles take place when we make them so: when we allow life events—even illness and tragedy—to help us discover the oneness of our soul.

I have never spoken with a patient, however sick, who has not felt that in some way his illness has presented him with the opportunity for a miracle. Perhaps a crisis has resulted in a rediscovered love; the forgiveness of a past transgression; a new view of what life means; an insight into the relative unimportance of local, mechanical living; or a new commitment to wellness.

Oneness and "Now What?"

We live in a do-it-yourself culture with an emphasis on the *do*. Such terms as adjusting, coping, adapting, and managing are common in our vocabulary. When we face a crisis, our instinct is to respond with "Quick! Now what do I do?"

During my pain, I became annoyed by the constant pressure I was putting on myself to "do something." "I've got to think of something to do," I kept saying. "Now what do I do?" Then, a coincidence happened that provided another oneness lesson.

At the same time that I was bedridden by the pain and immobility of my ever-worsening and -stiffening back, and as several doctors continued to diagnose my problem as a severe muscle sprain, my wife and I were having our home in Michigan rebricked. We had noticed that the harsh winter weather was causing some of the bricks to chip away from our house. I didn't know it then, but my house and my hips were both falling apart at the same time.

One afternoon, I heard a terrible crash. Hundreds of bricks came tumbling into my fireplace and thumping off the roof onto the ground. I looked out my second-story bedroom window and saw a workman sitting on the roof near where there used to be a chimney that he had just finished repairing after days of hard work. All of his effort was wasted. In fact, everything was worse than when he had started his repair. His eyes were closed, his head bowed, and his hands were resting on his knees as if he were in meditation.

"Are you all right?" I shouted.

After a pause, he answered, "I am. The chimney isn't. I mean it really is not. It's gone."

"Now what?" I asked. "What are you going to do now?"

"That's easy," he answered. "I just follow my usual sequence when these things happen. I swear, throw something, and then I do the most important thing. I sit down, shut up, and do nothing. If I sit down and do nothing long enough, something always happens or occurs to me. Somehow, everything resolves itself. It's just the way it is."

As I remember this bricklayer's words now, I think how often Patsy's principle reveals itself to us in our daily life. I never saw the bricklayer again, but months later, and when I was much sicker, I spoke with the manager of our brickwork. Everything was finished and the chimney was back in place stronger than ever. I envied the chimney and wished that I could be put back together so easily. "What happened to the guy who was there when the chimney fell?" I asked.

"Oh, I fired him," said the supervisor. "I found him just sitting there. When I asked him what happened, he said he had decided to become a house painter instead of a brick man. He said something told him to work in a different medium . . . something that didn't hurt when it fell on him. I guess he thought he was some kind of artist. He said he found a new way to make a living."

I learned from this simple story that sometimes the best answer to "Now what?" is revealed by doing absolutely nothing. We keep trying to fix things "our way" rather than tune in to "the Way." When we feel pressured to achieve some form of closure, some immediate problem-solving strategy, it may be more helpful to be quiet and try to be open to the infinite options and clearer Way that might come to us if we don't scare them away by the intensity and urgency of our search.

I have followed the bricker-turned-painter philosophy. During the several crises of my illness, I learned to let my emotions go freely, but briefly, to do something physical such as throw something, break something, or just slam my hand on the bed. Then, I used the "sit down and shut up" technique. Many popular books suggest the use of imagery, meditation, and healing exercises as paths to healing. One of the best paths, however, is to stop trying, going, and doing and just "be." There is something about our oneness that will provide us with clues about strategies and coping techniques that we may not even think of when we are too busy doing. We can't hear us when we are too busy trying to do it ourselves.

One of the best books ever written about being sick is *The Magic Mountain*, by Thomas Mann. It is a book full of satire and metaphors about life in a sanitarium for the treatment of tuberculosis. The main character in this book is Hans Castorp, who says, "There are two ways to life: one is the regular, direct, and good way; the other is bad, it leads through death, and this is the way of genius."[7] The "regular" way is the problem-averse local life of the see-and-touch world. What Mann calls the "bad" way is the way of learning through crises and suffering. The genius we achieve through this is a higher level of knowing that gives meaning to all of the trials and tribulations of living. If we wait, listen, feel, and look for meaning and oneness rather than hurry, try, fear, and surrender, we can develop what Mann calls a "higher sanity."

Oneness and "So What?"

Once the panic of serious illness or crisis diminishes, as it always does, our questions turn from Why me? Why now? and Now what? to the ultimate question: So what? Why is there suffering? What possible purpose is served by ravaging illnesses such as cancer?

Early in my illness, I wondered why I had to have so much pain.

Certainly, I thought, God could have us work His will without the lesson of severe suffering. I felt punished unfairly. Then, another coincidence happened that provided answers from the new science finding of oneness.

I had gone to the first in a series of doctors who failed to diagnose my cancer. While sitting in the physician's waiting room, a woman walked into the room carrying a large basket, an old watering can, and a bag labeled "plant food." She smiled at me and the other patients and then knelt by one of the several plants.

"Well, how are you today?" she asked the plant. All of us felt a little uncomfortable, but we all smiled. At least on a theoretical level, we had all heard that plants grow better if you talk nicely to them. Not that we actually believed plants could listen and feel, but most of us at least believed that talking to plants is a prudent gardening tip.

The woman began to prune the plant. She would first stroke a few leaves, and ever so gently cut off a part of each plant. "It really hurts them and it hurts me, too. The other plants feel it. Can't you, my little plant friends?" asked the woman. We all definitely felt awkward by now, yet we all looked around waiting for the plants to answer. And each of us sitting in that waiting room winced with each clip of the pruning shears.

The plant woman continued her work without looking up. She placed each cut branch gently into a bag. As if talking only to herself and her plants, she continued. "But they wouldn't be alive, we wouldn't be alive, if we and they couldn't feel pain. Pain is one thing we all share. Pain reminds us of how alive and connected we really are. Nobody wants the pain of birth, but we need it to be here." Before she left, the woman said good-bye to each and every plant in the room.

After the woman left, I felt an added spurt of pain in my back, and realized that I had just been given the answer to "So what?" A part of our being "one" is pain and suffering, just as a part of the plant's growth also brought the pain of pruning. The pain of childbirth, the emotional ache of loss and separation, and the anguish of illness are all signs of life, common to all of us. Later in my illness and healing, while I lay in bed in my home on the side of my magic mountain, the Haleakala volcano in Maui, I learned that pain and disease are paths to Mann's higher sanity.

Proof That Plants Think

One of the patients in the waiting room looked puzzled as the plant lady left. She turned to the man beside her and asked, "You really don't think that plants think, do you?"

"Oh, I'm sure they think," said the man gently touching the plant next to his chair. "I'm just not sure that they know they think." He laughed and all of us in the waiting room felt the awkwardness of those times when we confront such cosmic issues.

Much of this confusion about thinking, consciousness, and knowing is related to our definition of consciousness. Consciousness is much more than the sum total of a human being's neurochemical connections. Consciousness is a system of coming into coherence and interaction as one with the world.

Consciousness in its most basic form helps us find a local order in our daily lives. *Uncommon consciousness* in tune with the "way it is" helps us find the higher sanity of the universal chaos that underlies the major challenges in our lives.

Ask any gardener. Plants flourish when they are nurtured, coddled, and treated as if they share a common life with us. Skilled gardeners seem to interact with their plants, much as the musician seems to become a part of his or her instrument. Professor Herbert Frolich at Liverpool University in England has done research demonstrating "biological coherence," or the fact that all living systems, including plants, are organized and responsive systems.[8] A type of resonance, like the vibrating of a tuning fork, takes place within living cells and results in a higher life order. This coherence is the strong attraction toward oneness. We all share living with everything. Plants, popcorn, bowling balls, elephants: We all share vibrations of coherence together.

If we were to take hundreds of tiny compasses and jiggle them on a table, their needles would point in every possible random direction. However, if we were to connect the compasses by passing invisible but real electromagnetic current through them, all of the needles would line up in the same direction: The compasses would become a coherent whole and behave as one. This organizing oneness (separate singular elements falling together into an organized system) is an established fact of science. Many scientists have identified this tendency toward oneness. Some of their findings include

- Plato's "higher realm," or the idea that perfect forms or wholes emerge from parts attracted to one another by a oneness force. (Plato said that a horse ends up looking like a horse because of a "horse oneness" force—or a horse is a horse . . . of course!)
- Seventeenth-century scientist Johannes Kepler (discoverer of the moon's gravity effect on earth) proposed the theory that the earth is an animated or energized whole resulting from an inherent energy that unites all of the separate aspects of the planet.
- Rupert Sheldrake's work on "morphic fields and morphogenesis" indicated the tendency of everything to move toward oneness.
- Herbert Frolich's biological coherence theory mentioned above.
- Physicist and mathematician Ilya Prigogine's 1977 Nobel Prize–winning theory of dissipative structures or organization growing out of apparent chemical chaos.
- Biologist James Lovelock's "Gaia factor," referring to earth itself exhibiting a living wholeness.
- Yale University neuroanatomist Harold Burr's 1940s work on what he called "holographic energy growth templates."
- Albert Einstein's proposal of the Bose-Einstein condensate theory through which separate entities resonate into one system.
- Roman Catholic priest and physical anthropologist Pierre Teilhard de Chardin's "radial energy," or the force that draws individual elements to a higher order he called the "omega point."
- Philosopher Ludwig von Bertalanffy's "systems theory" proposed in the first half of this century, which suggested that parts move toward a new and more complex whole.

These scientists and dozens of others have clearly established the pervasiveness of a tendency toward oneness.

The Omega Factor

The priest and scientist Pierre Teilhard de Chardin described the tendency toward oneness as the "omega point"[9] (omega is the last letter of the Greek alphabet and derives from the concepts of finality and greatness). Miracles and coincidences are examples of the omega factor, or the sudden emergence of a "meaningful one" out of many.

An example of the omega factor, or the power of oneness, is revealed when experimenters place several individual heart cells in a petri dish and observe each individual cell contracting independently. Like the "hundredth monkey" effect mentioned at the beginning of this chapter, when several cells are added to the dish, the cells suddenly fall into a synchronicity (an omega point is reached) and "coincidentally" begin to beat in a normal, collective pulse of a healthy whole heart. Similarly, a few separate ants placed in the sand will wander about aimlessly. As more ants are added, however, they self-organize into a working omega community.[10]

The omega factor is essential to making miracles because it provides the energy, however difficult to measure, that allows us to feel the power of our oneness. True healing always involves the omega factor and the emergence of a new whole.

The Glow of Life

German biophysicist Fritz Popp has measured an actual glow coming from plants that probably is related to photon radiation.[11] He thinks that this glowing plays a major role in plant cell regulation. I am certain that cancer is related to something gone astray in the process of cell regulation caused by something like a short circuit in an energy field. Cancer cells have broken free of the omega force and are each behaving as if they were a whole unto themselves. Pain may be the buzzing of this short circuiting of the omega force. If we had sufficiently sensitive instruments to access this realm of reality, we would be able to differentiate an unhealthy glow from the glow of wellness.

"If you think that a plant can glow with health, or even a patient, then you are really stepping away from science," one of my colleagues told me. "This glow you speak of is simply a coloration of a system of chlorophyll or hemoglobin in balance. Nothing more."

"I agree completely," I answered. "The glow of energy that I speak of is a tangible sign of a system coming into balance and becoming much more than the sum of its parts. Call it the evidence of a Bose-Einstein condensate." With that, my colleague shook his head in disbelief and walked away. Most medical doctors think only in terms of biology, not physics. This means that they spend their professional time in only one of several realms of reality.

Vibrating into Something

Had my colleague known his physics, he would have recognized that physicists have given the name Bose-Einstein condensate theory to the idea that systems tend to resonate into coherent wholes.[12] Lasers are a current-day application of "bosons," or particles named after physicist Jagadis Chandra Bose. These bosons can "lase" together by exploding into billions of photons that cause the "whole" laser light. A laser beam results from invisible energy elements condensing into a visible and powerful whole.

Put simply, the central idea of the theory of a Bose-Einstein condensate is that the many parts that compose a given system can vibrate together (condense) and find their omega point, becoming a whole, responsive system.[13]

Another example of a Bose-Einstein condensate is superconduction, which is the capacity of certain metals and alloys (such as cadmium, aluminum, and mercury) to conduct electrical current without resistance when cooled to very low temperatures. At such temperatures, an "invisible field" is created within and around the alloy, allowing it literally to levitate and hover without "spending" or losing energy in the process. Their whole function becomes condensed into something much more than the sum of their parts, and the "paranormal" event of levitation or flying takes place because the rules of the mechanical world (such as gravity and the burning of energy) are transcended.

Frolich's coherent systems and Popp's glow of life are examples of how the superconductor-like processes of the Bose-Einstein condensate theory are applicable to our everyday lives and can be seen as explanations of how plants, for example, become a whole, functioning, interacting system—much more than just a set of singular cells processing chlorophyll and conducting photosynthesis.

The "So what?" lesson of oneness is that the crises in our lives are ways in which we ourselves are "jiggled" or vibrated to a new, higher level oneness. Pain, illness, and life challenges are the pruning and trimming necessary for the growth of our soul. We have been given the gift of being able to interpret and give meaning to the tests and trials of our life, so in effect we can be our own gardeners, not just mechanics maintaining our daily functions.

Thinking Stuff

To regulate the terrible pain of cancer and its treatment and to help me deal with the pain of related surgeries for my diagnosis and treatment, I was placed on a machine that allowed me to push a morphine-release button. Every time I felt too much pain, I could press the button, and a powerful analgesic would be sent through my veins. The dosage is carefully regulated and calibrated so that only so much medicine can be given no matter how many times a patient pushes in pain.

I'm certain that there is a strong placebo effect from this machine. Sometimes, your push of pain does not result in any medicine being released because you have exceeded the prescribed dosage. You never really know when you are getting the real medicine, but just pushing seems to make you feel better.

I quickly discovered that the trick to dealing with this machine is to merge with the machine, getting into a rhythm of pushing and pain. If you "fight" the machine, by becoming angry or impatient with it, the machine becomes a burden instead of a help. If you interact with the machine, actually talk to it and encourage it to work with you and show it a respect for the work it can do, it can be a big help in pain reduction.

A classic experiment done by physicist John Wheeler illustrates how such machines as the pain-push machine might be "conscious" as defined by the concept of oneness and coherence. Wheeler set up an investigation through which a photon is given the "choice" to go through either of two slits in a screen. A photon is a quantum (stuff) of electromagnetic energy that demonstrates the principle of complementarity in that it is simultaneously both wave and particle, having no electrical charge or mass but possessing momentum and energy. Therefore, due to the principle of complementarity, a photon always has the option of being either particle or wave depending on what its environment calls for and, as Wheeler's study proves, on what the photon "chooses" to do.

When Wheeler placed particle detectors on the other side of the two-slitted screen, the photon behaved like a particle and followed a path through one of the two slits, making a direct hit on a particle detector.[14] If Wheeler placed a detector between the screen and the particle detectors, however, the photon "chose" to behave like a wave. It took a path through *both slits* at the same time, interfered with itself, and left a pattern of this interference on the detection screen. In Wheeler's experiment, then, the photon, at least on some level of reality, seems to "know" about its environment, anticipate what detectors and screens will be on the other side of the two-slit screen, adjust to the situation, make "decisions" about how to interact with the circumstances, and respond and adapt. In a way, the "photon stuff" thinks. It makes adjustments in its "lifestyle" depending on where it is living. Like my pain machine, the photon is capable of behaving in oneness with its world. I suggest that thinking is a process of being "one" with everything; it is an alertness, acknowledgment, adjustment, and interaction with the cosmos. In this sense, photons and all the "stuff" in the universe "think."

Talking to the Animals

As I pointed out earlier in my discussion of the elephants, a feeling of oneness with animals is a commonly accepted point of view among animal lovers. When I was unable to walk because of my cancer, I knew that now more than ever I *had* to walk. Pressure on my hips might help to recalcify my pelvic bones. However, I just did not have the energy or the will to endure the pain of pulling myself across the floor with my walker while suffering the draining side effects of my chemotherapy.

My golden retriever Hana (Hawaiian for spirit) would get up in the middle of the night and nudge me with her nose. She would not stop bothering me until I got up and forced myself to walk through our family-room-turned-hospital-room. She continued to prod me along through my pain step by small agonizing step with my walker. I thought at first that Hana wanted to go outside or wanted something to eat, but she would just follow behind me, nudging me along with her nose. She took me just a little farther every night. Part of the reason my hips grew back and I can walk is because of my relationship with Hana.

Hundreds of studies document the communication of humans with other species.[15] We have all heard stories of pets finding their way back home over remarkable distances. Author Bill Schul[16] describes the case of the collie dog Bobbie who became lost in Indiana when her family moved from Ohio to their new home in Oregon. The family searched for Bobbie for hours, but had to move on. Three months later, Bobbie showed up at the doorstep of the family's home in Oregon.[17]

This story was so stunning that it appeared in several newspapers. A subsequent check of the story was conducted, and evidence was found of several families caring for Bobbie during her pilgrimage. A direct route from Indiana to the family's home in Oregon could be retraced by the reports of people who had seen and cared for the dog. Bobbie had taken the most direct and reasonable cross-country route.

The idea that we share a consciousness with animals, plants, and even "things" can change the way we treat our world. If we honor our oneness with the cosmos, we will preserve and respect the earth's resources and recognize our natural bond with everything in and on it. The way to miracles is through unity, not control. New science proves that we don't think alone; we just think we are alone, and we are mistaken.

Making It with a Machine

I could feel the morphine machine beginning to adjust with me. It seemed to buzz on its own, signaling a small release of painkiller just before my pain worsened. Any painkiller is most effective before an escalation of the pain, and the machine is programmed to release analgesic even when the patient does not push for it. The amazing fact is that, when I stopped pushing for pain relief, the machine began to do the pushing for me! It perfectly anticipated my pain and became a part of me rather than a machine working on me. For two days, I experienced the relief of spurts of pain medication whenever I needed it, but not once did I actually push the button.

"I can see you are really hurting, but the painkiller seems to be helping," said Dr. Death Vader. "You've been pushing the button almost every half hour even through the night."

"No I haven't," I said. "Besides, you know that I have been sleeping through the night."

"Don't be silly. Someone pushed the button, and we don't do it," insisted Dr. Vader. "The machine didn't do it itself."

"I think the machine and I struck a bargain and it took over for me," I said. "I think it started to make some decisions with and for me. It sort of sensed me."

"Right," said Dr. Vader, as he busily wrote a note that no doubt indicated that my new level of reality was unfamiliar to him and, therefore, pathological.

Remember the bricks that were chipping away outside my home? By coincidence, they were doing so at exactly the same time that my own hip bones were chipping away. The "stuff" of my house was reflecting what was happening with the "stuff" of my body. As strange as such examples may seem to you, please consider the scientific proof presented in this book that illustrates that there is no such thing as separateness.

Feel your environment. Feel your connection to the bricks, the plants, the animals, and the machines all around you. We think that the electrons of a chair are not exactly the same electrons within our own body and brain. We are wrong. An electron is an electron, whether it is in a brick or a bone. We need not feel isolated from one another or from any element of our world. We are everywhere and a part of everything.

Oneness and the Science of Prayer

Whenever I discuss the "science" of prayer, my audiences divide immediately into particles (lumps) and waves (jumps). About half of the audience becomes resistant, uncomfortable, and even angry. They are operating from a particle-oriented, here-and-now view of the world. Prayer to them is at best a religious or superstitious ritual that probably does no harm but certainly does no tangible good.

The wave, or energy jump, half of the audience sees a magical, spiritual, powerful quality to prayer and praying. Some wave people become angry when I start to talk about scientific research relating to prayer. They feel that scientific inquiry into prayer violates the sanctity of prayer.

The principle of uncertainty reminds us that if we take strictly a concrete, research orientation to praying, we ignore the spiritual and personal power of prayer. Conversely, if we mystify prayer by viewing it as something that cannot be studied, analyzed, or learned from, we neglect one of the most remarkable of all scientific facts: As predicted by faith and proven by the scientific principles of nonlocality and oneness, *prayer works!* The principle of complementarity teaches that *both* science and religion are correct in what they teach us, and that both can simultaneously explain the power of prayer.

Prayer from and for the Heart

In 1988—the same year that I first became sick—an important and carefully done study on the power of prayer was published by cardiologist Randolph Byrd.[18] This study met the most stringent of guidelines for careful medical research.

In Byrd's ten-month study, a computer randomly selected 192 patients admitted to a coronary unit at the San Francisco Hospital as the unknowing recipients of the prayers of regular home prayer meetings taking place throughout the United States. Another 201 patients were not so assigned. Neither the patients, nurses, doctors, nor families of the patients knew which group was being prayed for. Roman Catholic and Protestant groups from around the country were recruited to pray for the members of the "prayer recipient" group. The home prayer groups were given only the names of the patients, a few details about the medical condition of the patients, and were told to pray in any way they chose but to pray each day. Each patient in the prayer-recipient group had between five and seven people throughout the country praying for him or her every day.

The results of this study were stunning. The prayer recipients were five times less likely than the unremembered group to require antibiotics and three times less likely to develop complications. None of the prayed-for group required a life-support system, and fewer (although not a statistically significant number) died. (One reason why the least statistically significant finding was in the area of survival may rest with Patsy's principle. Death and disease are natural and "the Way" or "Thy Will." If everyone who is prayed for lived forever, we would all die of overcrowding. There is "a Way" beyond our comprehension, and our prayers are effective only within "the Way," not as demands for "our way.")

Dr. William Nolan is a physician who attempts to expose false claims of faith healing and miracles in medicine. Of Byrd's study, however, he writes, "It sounds like this study will stand up to scrutiny . . . maybe we doctors ought to be writing on our order sheets, 'Pray three times a day.' If it works, it works."[19]

I can state unequivocally from my own MM group study and my personal experiences through my disease and treatment that prayer works and we can prove it! If we accept the findings of new science, including the key principles of nonlocality and oneness, then the power of prayer and healing at a distance are easy facts to accept and understand.

How to Pray the Right Way

For more than ten years, a research group called Spindrift has been doing careful, replicated, scientific studies of prayer.[20] The word *spindrift* comes from the Scottish word used to describe sea spray driven by the wind and waves. It is a perfect name to illustrate the oneness I have been stressing in this chapter because it symbolizes the universal connection of the forces of nature.

Below are ten recommendations that I have formulated, based on the Spindrift research, for celebrating the miracle-making power of our oneness through the power of prayer.

The Ten Commandments of Prayer

1. Because every person shares oneness with God, every person has divine attributes. The Spindrift studies showed that the power of prayer is available to anyone and everyone. It is not a special gift of only a few "healers." The people who prayed in the Spindrift studies were common people with no special qualifications other than their beliefs in our oneness. Furthermore, neither the Catholics nor the Protestants were proven to be superior prayers in Byrd's prayer study.

2. Prayer works. The Spindrift studies involved two groups of

rye seeds growing in the same container cared for in exactly the same manner. A string down the middle of the container divided the seeds. One set of seeds was prayed for, and the other was not. The prayed-for side flourished much more than the side not prayed for. No matter how many times this study was repeated, the results were the same. Prayed-for seeds survive and prosper more than not-prayed-for seeds. This study also supports my contention of interaction between people and plants and all of the stuff in the world.

3. Prayer works even better at times of crisis. When the Spindrift researchers added salt water to stress all of the rye seeds in the container, the prayed-for seeds did *even better* than in the first studies of unstressed seeds!

4. Prayer works better and better the worse and worse things seem to get. When researchers added even more salt water to the container, they discovered that the saltier the solution, the stronger and more positive the effect of prayer. This finding is corroborated in the medical world: All doctors know that the stronger the patient's pain, the more powerful the positive effect of a placebo, or false pill. True faith combined with the challenge of severe stress seems to result in the omega point I mentioned earlier, and the power of our oneness is magnified.

5. Prayer works for anyone and anything. The Spindrift group switched from studying rye seeds to studying soybeans and tried changing the stressors to high or low temperature and more or less humidity. No matter what was being prayed for, the more severe the stress, the stronger the effect of the prayer. This finding supports my contention that pain and chaos are the jigglers, or stimulants, of the oneness and coherence illustrated by the Bose-Einstein condensate theory.

6. The more one prays, the more powerful the prayer. The Spindrift researchers wondered if more prayer led to better results. They divided the seeds and varied the time the seeds were prayed for. When the time prayed was doubled, the positive effect on the seeds doubled as well.

7. Prayer is more powerful if we know who and what we are praying for. When the people praying were kept uninformed about the nature of the seeds being prayed for, there was a drastic decrease in the effect of praying. This supports my

point about the role of observer participantcy or "what you see makes what you get." Seeing—or at least having an image of the prayer target—increases our prayer efficiency and helps us hit and heal our target.

8. Practiced prayer makes more perfect prayer. Some people who pray are indeed more effective than others. The Spindrift researchers compared the effectiveness on various seeds of more and less practiced prayers. The more one prays, the more powerful one's prayers become. This prayer proficiency factor may be due to the influence of the principles of observer participantcy and the omega point power generated by reaching a critical mass of prayer power. If you need some prayer help in an emergency, call in someone who has kept in practice. Panic prayer by the prayer novice turning to God for emergency help should be supplemented by a more experienced spiritual communicator.

9. Prayer works on everything from the most simple aspect of life to the most complex systems in the universe. No matter how many seeds were involved in the Spindrift research, the power of prayer was strong and could not be overwhelmed by the number of seeds prayed for. The earth itself is not too complex to respond to our prayers: Ecologists and environmentalists would be well advised not only to recycle and conserve but also to pray for the well-being of our planet.

10. Prayer for "Thy will" rather than "my will" is the most effective prayer. In nondirected "Thy will" prayer, the person praying does not attempt to tell the universe what to do. *Modern approaches that emphasize visualization and imagery techniques may be misguided.* In the Spindrift study of the differences between directed imagery type of prayer and prayer for God to work His will, the more nondirected, accepting approach had the most powerful effect on the seeds.

When we pray, we do not "bounce energy" off some type of cosmic satellite. When we pray, we pray *with* and not *to* God and we pray as one with each other and with God. Prayer is immediate, spontaneous, and it transcends time and space. People in Byrd's study who lived closer to the heart patients did not have a more positive effect than people who lived a country away.

When I was dying, there were several prayer groups praying for me. I could feel them and I could sometimes see them. I could see and feel a group of nurses with hands joined, heads lowered, praying that the right thing would happen for me. (I wonder if we bow our heads in prayer not only in reverence but as a symbolic way to "stand out less" and to be a more humble part of humanity's oneness.) I could see the entire congregation of churches in cities where my friends lived praying aloud in unison that "Thy will" would be done for me. Like Dr. Dossey's blind patient whom I mentioned earlier who could "see" so clearly, I too could "see" or sense my mother's, brother's, and all of my family's prayers, both around my bed and from across the country. I could "hear" the participants at a major scientific meeting being asked for a moment of silence for me. I could hear the music of a small band composed of my friends as they attempted to send the vibrations of oneness to me when I needed harmony so much. If any of those powerful people who prayed for me are reading this, please know that your prayers worked. I am praying for you, too.

Don't Give Orders to the Universe: Let the Universe Order You

Pray for oneness and "Thy will," and your prayers will always be answered. A prayer for Thy will is a prayer for "the way" of nature, for Patsy's "just the way it is."

When you stop giving orders to the cosmos and start letting the cosmos reveal its order to and through you, you will see that a cosmic magic is at work on many levels at the same time. This is why miracles seem to pop up in the most unlikely places at the least-expected moment. As you will discover in chapter 7, your chances for catching a miracle are greatly increased once you combine an understanding of oneness with the next sacred secret of science: the existence of multiple realms of reality.

NOTES

1. L. Watson, *Lifetide: The Biology of Consciousness* (New York: Simon & Schuster, 1980).
2. The "hundredth monkey phenomenon" has been described in science classes throughout the country. The typical reaction by scientists and students alike is the "Helmholtzian position" that, even if it is true, they refuse to believe it.

3. Erwin Schrödinger. *What Is Life? and Mind and Matter* (London: Cambridge University Press, 1969), 133.

4. *Ibid.*, 140

5. This is a remarkable little booklet that allows children and adults to physically experience the scale of the universe through the use of common household objects. One actually "feels" the size of the cosmos by following the assignments in this pamphlet. See Guy Ottewell, *The Thousand-Yard Model* (Greenville, SC: Furman University Press, 1989).

6. Larry Dossey is a leader in the application of the laws of new science to medicine. See his ground-breaking book, *Space, Time, and Medicine* (Boston: New Science Library, 1982), 176.

7. Thomas Mann, *The Magic Mountain* (New York: Vintage Books, 1969), 725.

8. Herbert Frolich, "Coherent Excitations in Active Biological Systems," in *Modern Bioelectrochemistry*, ed. F. Gutman and H. Keyzer (New York: Plenum, 1986).

9. P. Teilhard de Chardin, *The Phenomenon of Man* (New York: Harper & Row, 1959), 65.

10. E. Jantsch, *The Self-Organizing Universe* (New York: Pergamon Press, 1980).

11. Fritz Albert Popp et al. "Physical Aspects of Biophotons," *Experiences* 44 (1977).

12. Sir Jagadis Chandra Bose was an Indian physicist and plant physiologist who did his work in the 1920s and 1930s.

13. Bose-Einstein condensates are similar to the harmonics when one hears a car horn. Two pitches are combined so that one sound results. The sound not only behaves and sounds like one sound but it actually "becomes" one sound. A technical explanation of such a phenomenon as applied to the human brain is found in C. I. J. M. Stuart et al., "Mixed Brain Dynamics: Neural Memory as a Macroscopic Ordered State," *Foundations of Physics* 9, nos. 3–4 (1979).

14. Described in John Archibald Wheeler, "Beyond the Black Hole," in *Some Strangeness in the Proportion*, ed. Harry Woolf (Reading, MA: Addison-Wesley, 1980).

15. See the work of biologist Lyall Watson, *Gifts of Unknown Things* (New York: Simon & Schuster, 1986). In this book, Dr. Watson describes numerous examples of miracles taking place in the interaction between humans and animals.

16. Bill Schul, *The Psychic Power of Animals* (New York: Fawcett, 1977).

17. *Ibid.*, 52.

18. Randolph C. Byrd, "Positive Therapeutic Effects of Intercessory

Prayer in a Coronary Care Unit Population," *Southern Medical Journal* 81, no. 7 (1988): 826–829.

19. Quoted in Howard Wolinsky, "Prayers Do Aid Sick, Study Finds," *Chicago Sun-Times,* Jan. 26, 1986, 30.

20. Described in the book by Robert Owen, *Qualitative Research: The Early Years* (Salem, OR: Grayhaven Books, 1988). More information on the Spindrift organization can be obtained by writing to Spindrift, 2407 La Jolla Drive NW, Salem, OR 97304.

7
REALMS OF REALITY

The Cure for Divinity Dyslexia

Einstein's space is no closer to reality than Van Gogh's sky.

—ARTHUR KOESTLER

I'm astounded by people who want to "know" the universe when it's hard enough to find your way around Chinatown.

—WOODY ALLEN

Reality is a crutch for people who can't cope with drugs.

—LILY TOMLIN

Doctors' Domain Dyslexia

My cancer was spreading. It was eating away most of my pelvic bone. The pain was shifting from the middle of my upper back to my hips, and I felt weak, nauseated, and afraid. I could do little more than shuffle from my wheelchair to a hospital bed that my wife had rented and placed in our family room. "We're keeping you a part of us. You're not going to a bedroom. You'll stay here in the family room until you get better. We're going to do together everything that we have always done," said my wife.

Since that 8/8/88 day, I had become a near invalid, yet doctor after doctor dismissed my illness as a "serious back strain and sprain." Every doctor made the same three mistakes that constitute what I call "domain dyslexia." Every doctor believed that valid measurements would come only through their mechanical instruments, that there was one, local cause for every mechanically detected effect, and that there is only one reality explainable by one grand theory of everything. Anything that didn't fit that criteria was labeled "impossible." Like the person with a reading disability, the doctors could not read the complete story of my illness because *they were blind to the symbols and rules of the language of other realities.*

Psychologist Lawrence LeShan and physicist Henry Margenau write, "The assumption that there is one 'true' definition of all reality is outworn. . . . There is no contradiction between different valid systems of explanation—different valid realities. But they are profoundly different."[1] You have already read how the laws of oneness and observer participantcy operate in "creating reality." Unfortunately, the doctors I consulted were observing only one realm of reality. The famous medical statement "spontaneous remission," which literally means a quick stop, is the doctors' attempt to use the language of this one reality realm to explain a realm of miracles that far transcends the local laws of their mechanical training.

Having Fleas and Worms at the Same Time

In spite of my severe pain, my wife and I together took our dog, Hana, to the veterinarian. The dog had been sluggish, yet she was eating more than ever. I was in such pain that I could only sit in the waiting room while my wife pulled Hana into the veterinarian's examination room and hoisted her reluctant body onto the table. I had suspected that Hana's unusual appetite indicated that she might have worms in her intestines. Every dog owner knows of this disgusting problem.

When my wife and the veterinarian came to the waiting room with Hana, he said, "She has fleas."

"But I thought for sure that she had worms," I answered.

"She has worms, too," he answered. "Dogs can have worms and fleas at the same time."

For some reason, this simple statement had a profound effect on me. Like my doctors, I had accepted the local reality of searching for the *one cause* leading directly to my pain and sickness. No one "thought to think" that I might be sick on an entirely different level of reality that could not be measured by blood tests or by standard X ray (all of which had come out negative). With this more open approach to my condition, we set out to find doctors of different domains.

The Beginning of Domain Hopping

My first doctor in August and September of 1988 was a holistic doctor. This particular physician claimed to have expertise in the domain of treating the "whole" patient. He ran the standard tests and pronounced that I had a sprained back.

I told him that I felt much too sick to be suffering from just a bad back. He answered, "I've had a bad back myself. They can be much worse than you think. Let me prove my point through accupressure." He pushed at a secret point just inside my lower ribs, and pain shot through my body from my forehead to my groin. I almost fell off the examining table.

"See," he said, seeming pleased. "That's clearly a back sprain." He walked out of the room and brought back sample medications given him by a drug salesman. "These are pain pills for your back. [I wondered why the pills were "for my back" and not for "all of me."] Take these three times a day, meditate, and use guided imagery and relaxation. Watch your diet, too."

This doctor called himself holistic because he prescribed vitamins and motivational tapes for his patients. He, in fact, was as limited in his view of one reality as any other doctor I saw. His holism was simply a different version of mechanical medicine. There is no evidence in any research journal or at any medical center in the world that meditation, positive attitude, touch, vitamins, or specific guided imagery cures any disease, but holism advocates assert that such approaches are proven effective by the absence of disproof. In my case, this doctor's false holism and failure to read other realities almost killed me.

The pain was so severe that, when I traveled to my lectures, I flew across the country standing up to prevent becoming trapped in my airplane seat and suffering the agonizing rigidity that inevitably would set in. I could not move on the stage as I addressed my audiences, and even as I talked, I thought and worried about my condition.

I wondered how a back could "be bad." We all have the best backs there are. Pain signals that a readjustment is taking place, not that our back has turned evil. I worry about calling the parts of our body that need our help bad names. These parts are listening. I felt that my back must feel insulted just when I needed it to be cooperating with me the most.

In an attempt at domain hopping, I thought that body movement exercises might help. I bought a videotape on "back therapy" and I began my own therapy for a back injury. The doctor on the tape said, "First, lie down on the floor." I couldn't do it. The pain was too severe and my pelvis would not allow me to move to that position. That tape has never moved beyond the first inches on my videotape player.

I tried hopping domains by reading several different books on back pain. Each book had its own solution within its own reality realm. Not one mentioned the possibility of illness in the realm of the energy of the cell. Nor did any author, holistic or otherwise, *combine* realms to discover the various domains in which I was suffering.

During this time, ironically, I toured several cities lecturing on my book titled *Super Immunity: Master Your Emotions and Improve Your Health*. I was in agony myself, yet I was lecturing on the immune system that, unknown to me at that time, was in my case full of cancer. "If the audience only knew," I thought one evening in the middle of a lecture in New York. "The great expert on wellness is as sick as a dog."

"A dog!" In that instant I remembered. "Fleas and worms. Hana had fleas and worms. I've been trying to prove whether or not my back is sick, but I might have something else in addition to my back problem. It's not that I do not have a sprained back, but maybe I also have some form of flu. It's been going around lately." Thus began a parade to other realm specialists who put me in more pain and totally missed my diagnosis of potentially terminal cancer. The realization that there might be more than one cause for my suffering would eventually lead me to doctors who would help me, but at this time I was still trapped by the restrictive realities of "specialists" who saw only their own reality as "special."

The Five Realms

Before going further into the problem of reality realm dyslexia and how it affected my journey through illness, I'd like to share with you the science secret of five realms of reality. As I pointed out in chapter 5 where I described scientist John White's seven realms of the spirit, there are an infinite number of ways to classify the realities. The five realms presented here can serve as an initial guide for adventuring out into your own new realms, but they are gateways, not destinations. I hope you will remember each of these realms in your own daily life and not suffer the pain (as I did) of overlooking realms that could hold the answers to your own life problems.

Psychologist LeShan and physicist Margenau have described "five realms of experience,"[2] and I have modified their classification based on my own work with the MMs and my own illness and healing. Each realm involves a different way of measuring and knowing our universe. It is important to bear in mind that one realm is not more "real" than another, even though we have been taught that there is only one "right" reality.

Most psychologists view with suspicion people who talk about reality in the plural. *The ultimate pathology, however, is becoming trapped in one reality or trying to apply the rules of one reality to all others.* The reality of our childhood interactions with our parents is not always the best realm for relating to your parents as an adult, for example. Being stuck in one reality almost killed me. In chapter 4, I mentioned the value of being "abnormal" and "maladjusted" in terms of the traditional psychological definition of these terms. One way to ensure that you remain "abnormally healthy" is to reject the normalcy of seeing only one local, mechanical reality in everyday living.

When my son Roger was very young, we knew that he had a serious learning and reading problem. He was bright and alert, yet he was not learning to read. One day, when he saw a sign written in Japanese, he asked what it said. When I told him it was in another language, he began to cry. "Then I can't see one whole world," he said. The whole world of written letters appears to him to be a strange language.

Precisely because of his reading disability, however, Roger is able to see and know things that few of us will ever see or know. He crosses the boundaries between the realms of reality much better than most of us and has a creativity that amazes us. He does not impose the reality of the written word on the reality of the sound of music, for he would not be able to "read" notes. Instead, he feels and becomes a part of the music.

When Roger was in kindergarten, the other children were already far ahead of him in learning the alphabet. Fortunately for Roger, he had one of those rare teachers who works with learning disabilities by overcoming the teaching disability of instructing only in one realm of reality. This teacher sent Roger home with one of his few school successes.

"Look, Dad," said Roger. "I got an award. I wrote the right number for how many planets there are, and I was the winner."

"How many did you know?" I asked, suspicious because Roger had never read anything about our solar system and could not write legible numbers. "I guessed the number eight," he answered proudly.

"But there are nine planets, Roger," I said.

"I know that now, Dad. But eight was the only number I could write that I wouldn't write backward or upside down. The number eight is always right, and I was more right than they were!"

As you already know, the number eight "coincidentally" recurs continually in my family's life. In numerology, the number eight represents total immersion in all levels of the world. For example, it represents

- The "eight gifts of the yoga *siddhis*," each of which is related to a freedom from the constrictions of one level of reality.
- Eight represents "new life" or a new beginning.
- In music composition, an octave is composed of eight notes and every eighth note merges into unison with its counterparts.
- Shamans suggest that a man's body has seven orifices, but a woman has an eighth through which we are born.
- The number eight lying on its side represents infinity.
- Christians consider the number eight as representative of life after death or rebirth.
- Eight is the first cube number and thus represents a new dimension of mathematics.

The number eight would become even more significant for me and my family when I was in the deepest throes of my illness. Numbers that seem to reappear are often involved in the significant coincidences of our life.[3]

As my son Roger's school experience illustrates, no one is ever "completely right." The definition of what is right, or correct, varies depending on how we choose to understand our cosmos. Which realm we select is up to us at any given time. If one realm doesn't give us freedom or a sense of direction and well-being, we can select or combine them until we arrive at a reality that works for us.

Reality Realm Number One: The World of the Tiny and the Quick

One realm of reality that we have already discussed is the quantum world of the very, very small going very, very fast. This reality was proposed early in this century, and as you have seen, many of its concepts help us understand much about our living from an entirely different point of view.

The rules and measurements of this reality are quite different than those that we are used to. For example, in the see-and-touch domain (LeShan and Margenau's "third realm") the term *vacuum* represents complete emptiness and nothingness. In quantum reality, however, a vacuum is everything, including mass and energy, charge and spin, and such quantum "stuff" as relationships and correlations.[4] American physicist David Finkelstein wrote, "A general theory of the vacuum is thus a theory of everything."[5] British physicists Tony Hey and Patrick Walters describe the quantum vacuum as " 'bubbling soup' of virtual particle/antiparticle pairs."[6]

One drawback of a life led only in the see-and-touch realm is that the threat of us ultimately becoming a vacuum and a dread of final nothingness always hangs over our heads. The quantum world of reality, however, holds the promise of ultimate "everythingness."

Reality Realm Number Two: The World of the Huge and the Whizzing

Before the year 1916 and the impact of Albert Einstein's work, space was seen not only as an empty vacuum but also as being infinite. Some of us still believe that we live here on planet earth surrounded by a vast emptiness that goes on forever, ruled over by a God who sits somewhere outside all of this running everything. Philosopher Baruch Spinoza, the founder of pantheism (the concept of the presence of God in everything and in each of us), wrote that separateness from God is impossible. He wrote, "The general laws of nature which govern and determine all phenomena are nothing but the eternal decrees of God which always entail eternal truth and necessity."[7]

When Albert Einstein was asked if he believed in God, he answered, "I believe in the God of Spinoza." He was referring to the fact that his studies had revealed the *presence* of God in everything in the universe rather than an *image* of a God who sits outside a universe that He impulsively alters at will while He allows it to spiral into nothingness.

Philosopher Giordano Bruno, who preceded Spinoza, wrote, "God is not an external intelligence, rolling around and leading around; it is more worthy of Him to be the internal principle of motion, which is His own nature, His own appearance, His own soul."[8] Bruno was martyred for his rational view of God: He was burned at the stake. Spinoza was excommunicated for his form of spirituality. Both of these great philosophers were victims of the clash between rationalism and faith and a clinging to a one-reality view.

The fates of Spinoza and Bruno illustrate a long-standing intolerance of seeing the divine in the "real" world. If we cannot embrace the existence of several realms and a divinity that crosses through multiple realities, we are left with the illusion of having to choose between "certain fact" or "blind faith."

As an example of multiple ways of seeing reality, the see-and-touch level of reality suggests that two perfectly parallel lines extended through space would go on "forever" and never meet. A straight line is seen as the shortest distance between two points. Realm-hopper Albert Einstein's theory of general relativity shook this conviction by proving that space and time could be one and the same, that space only "looked" infinite, that "curvedness" was a more direct route through the cosmos than a straight line, and that two parallel lines could eventually merge. Once Einstein catapulted us into the discovery of this new realm of reality, it became clear that mechanical rules were no longer the only rules of the cosmos.

More than anything else, Einstein taught us that Spinoza and Baruch were correct in finding divinity on many levels of our living. He would often lecture about the existence of multiple dimensions of our experiences by using the example of a caterpillar that knows only one dimension, forward and backward. As that caterpillar crawls along the surface of a large ball, it thinks that it is going in a straight line. The caterpillar would become aware of another dimension of reality only if it were to return to its caterpillar starting blocks and discover that it had been there before.

My own illness and surviving near death constituted my own rediscovery of me: where I come from and where I am going. When a crisis causes a level of introspection that leads you smack into *you*, you learn much about how many different realities there are.

One of the young MMs who was suffering from leukemia made her own Einsteinian formula that illustrates the influence of multiple realities. She said, "Dr. Pearsall, I have a new formula for you. Einstein said that energy is equal to mass multiplied by the speed of light squared, or $e = mc^2$. For me, e stands for enjoyment and the m stands for the meaning we give to our life. The c^2 stands for many ways to see the cosmos. So for me, $e = mc^2$ means the enjoyment of our life is equal to the meaning we see in our life and the power of many levels of the cosmos. Do you think I should write a book about my form of relativity?"

The world of the very, very big going very, very fast proves that space and time are the same and that they are not fixed forever. Space and time are "bendable," and if we could go fast enough, we could go backward in time and become younger and younger. The local, linear laws of our daily experience do not work well in the big whizzing world of Einstein.

Reality Realm Number Three: The World of Me and It

LeShan and Margenau refer to a third realm of reality as the see-and-touch world. We experience this world as the "real" world we live in; the world of "me" doing "things" with "stuff." This is the

Newtonian world of predictable mechanical rules. Time goes only forward, effect follows cause, everything is measurable, and the world is local or here and now.

We tend to be stuck in this third realm of "me and it." I broke free of this realm to discover the energies from the quantum and cosmic realms that also influenced my illness and healing. In doing so, I discovered, like the MM mentioned earlier, the miracle of joy and hope that springs from many meanings rather than one way of knowing.

Even our religions remain trapped in this one level of reality when they attempt to make God into an anthromorphic image operating by one set of simple laws. When a simple, mechanical law is "broken," we think that a miracle has taken place.

Thomas Aquinas defined a miracle as something "done by divine power apart from the order generally followed in things." By "generally followed in things," he meant the here-and-now, see-and-touch world. I have defined a miracle as a meaningful coincidence that suddenly exposes the presence of several differing realities, all operating simultaneously under the infinite realities of God. Miracles are not examples of rule breaking; they are evidence of the power of differing rules. As I pointed out in chapter 3, God does not have to break His own rules to prove His existence; the magnificence of the multiple workings of the cosmos is evidence enough.[9]

Reality Realm Number Four: The World of Our Interpretation

This realm of reality is the realm of the social sciences and the arts. Humankind has formulated a system of thinking and being in the world that is referred to as "culture." Culture is the realm of reality that we use to give meaning to our behavior.

During my training as a psychologist, I learned that much of this level of reality is based on a mechanical view of living. Sigmund Freud's structure of the personality, his concept of the id, and the linear view of our progression and regression through unfolding life stages and conflicts of our psychosexual development are all based on a Newtonian model of the human psyche. The traditional question of the psychotherapist—"Why?"—is based on the cause-and-effect assumption so basic to psychodynamics.

When a psychiatrist was called to help me cope with my depression after I was told I was going to die, I wondered what he would have to say. As I expected, he asked the "Why?" question. I responded that I was totally involved in this crisis, that depression was a key emotion that was not destructive, and that "Tell me everything about how you are feeling right now" would have been a better orientation than "Why are you depressed?"

The psychiatrist assumed that my depression was caused by my reaction to my diagnosis: a simple one cause and one effect. He failed to see that I was wrestling—as everyone who confronts their mortality does in their own way—with cosmic and quantum issues that I had never before dealt with on such a personal level. Anatole Broyard, former *New York Times* book critic and editor, recently died of cancer. In his last essay about facing mortality, he wrote of "the wonder, terror and exaltation of being on the edge of being."[10] I was feeling this terror of the forced insight of impending death, and my depression was one dimension of that experience. Rather than distract me from life, my fear and pain actually kindled my need to reflect on the many levels of existence.

Art and music also exist in the "interpretive" realm of reality. They cannot be explained in purely mechanical terms; in fact they require various rules from all of the realms of reality. The rules of one realm are not always exclusive to that realm. This is why we can feel a sculpture of Michelangelo, almost hear a portrait by Goya speaking to us, talk of the "color" of harmonic tones or "notes" of color in a painting, see extraordinarily elaborate patterns of the music of Mozart, and even read the almost mathematical patterns of Bach's music, of whom it is said that he spoke in mathematics to God.

When I was in intensive care, unable to see or move, I learned to "see" thunder. The sensation was not symbolic. I actually visualized thunder. I heard it, but I also could see it as an image that is beyond words.

In the see-and-touch world, we can only hear thunder and see lightning. In the interpretive realm, however, we do not have to be limited by the firing of neurons that stimulate one area of the brain. Like miracle maker Helen Keller, we can become "sensuists" and take joy in a sensual world unlimited by the physical body. We can use our natural ability for synesthesia or merging and crossing-over of the senses.

Reality Realm Number Five: The World of the Spirit

This realm of reality is the reality of our inner and personal world. It is what we feel and believe about everything that happens to us. The spiritual domain is the realm of our communication with everything and everyone free of time and space. Much of what we call paranormal, or psi phenomena, occurs on this level. We are engaging this level of reality when we sense the meaning of coincidences and make our everyday miracles. We cannot touch the "stuff" of the spiritual world, but it is as real in its own domain as a chair is in the see-and-touch world, the speed of light in the cosmic world, simultaneity in the quantum world, and a symphonic work in the interpretive world.

The domain of the spirit, like all of the realms of reality, correlates with findings in cosmic and quantum science. In all of the research done on paranormal events such as remote seeing, predicting the future, and sensing the presence of others, there is absolutely no finding that violates the most firmly established laws of science as described in this book,[11] yet scientists have the most trouble accepting this realm of reality.

The realms of science and spirituality clash when we attempt to explain such phenomena as telepathy, clairvoyance, and precognition using the laws of the see-and-touch reality exclusively. As you have already seen in previous chapters, nonlocality, or simultaneity and action at a distance, is a proven fact. Paranormal events are entitled to the same serious examination and application of new science rules as phenomena that occur on the see-and-touch level.

In the play *The Search for Intelligent Life in the Universe*, the bag lady played by Lily Tomlin laments, "Reality is only a collective hunch." One big "hunch" will never provide us with all of the answers. We will never have and we do not need one big theory to explain everything. A key step in making miracles and in understanding the meaningful coincidences and synchronicities of our lives is to acknowledge the existence of the five realms of reality outlined here and to accept many different guesses about our many ways of experiencing our lives.

My Journey Through the Realms of Reality

I began my journey through the realms of reality with my futile visit
to the holistic doctor mentioned earlier. I then saw a neurologist who
was sure that I had a slipped disk. He ordered an MRI, or a magnetic
resonance imaging, test that would detect such a problem. When I
went for the appointment, I asked whether the fact that I had had
two prior retinal detachments corrected by the placement of metal
clips in my eyes would constitute a risk to my vision. The technician
matter-of-factly handed me a pamphlet that warned that I might go
blind if I had this test. The test was never done.

As my pain worsened, I sought the opinion of a physiatrist, a
doctor specializing in back pain. As I limped into his office, he
said, "Sure looks like a bad back to me." I thought, "My poor back.
Everyone keeps telling it how 'bad' it is."

The doctor examined me. He asked me to bend, but I could
barely lean forward. He ordered spinal X rays designed to detect a
fracture (but not the type of X ray that could detect the lymphatic
tumor that was eating my bones away), but said he was certain that
"nothing is broken. You just have a sprained back." He gave me
several exercises to do and once again I was trapped in a see-and-
touch reality realm. Pain here, corrective counterpressure there
seemed to be the approach.

I returned home, but the pain worsened. I went back to the
physiatrist. My wife and I expressed our sense of frustration and
despair at our continued failure to find relief, and the doctor responded, "I know, Paul, that you are a psychologist. But I would
like to tell you that I think a lot of your pain is in your mind. I read
your book *Superimmunity*. You said it: The strain of pain is mainly
in the brain. You're disappointed and depressed about the closing
of your clinic at the hospital. I know it; I work there too and they're
doing the same thing to me. You're just overburdened and broken.
In fact, you have turned to Jell-O. Just look at how you sit and walk.
You have to work yourself past this."

I was stunned. I certainly knew that psychological factors contributed to illness, but I also sensed that I was seriously ill. This
physician was switching realms on me. When his see-and-touch
model of diagnosis failed him, he tried unsuccessfully to apply his
mechanical rules to nonmechanical domains. In my doctor's

words, "They closed your clinic, so you have a burden that psychologically forced you to break." He was operating by a system of psychological hydraulics; pressure here, result there. However, the spiritual realm is not governed by hydraulic principles.

Mechanical systems are predictable, but other levels of reality are influenced by the principle of uncertainty. Local cause-and-effect systems are one directional, but other levels of reality operate by the principle of complementarity, or a mutual causation of alternative explanations. Looking for broken bone or strained muscle "masses" blinded the doctors from seeing disruptions of spiritual "energy."

I was weak and vulnerable, however, and my pain made me ready to cling to any explanation. "Now I've done it," I thought. "I've gone and caused my own illness. I've written about and lectured about such things, and now I've done it to myself." I went home and began to force myself through the pain to do the exercises that the physiatrist recommended. I screamed and cried, but I worked and worked. With every slight twist, my muscles ripped away from my cancer-eaten hips. After weeks of effort to solve my problem, I was much worse.

Because no doctor had yet found the realm of my suffering, they were not able to sense the magnitude of my pain. As a result, the prescriptions for painkilling drugs were extremely mild and had no effect on my pain. When I told my doctors of the ineffectiveness of the analgesics, they responded by suggesting that I "just take over-the-counter painkillers" and to "take as many as you need and see if that helps." My family cried and suffered with me as they offered sincere but useless suggestions to lessen my pain such as "take a warm bath" or "how about sleeping on a more firm mattress" or "try a heating pad." My wife would try to hold me and offer the comfort of her own warmth, but the slightest touch sent pain searing through my hips. A loving embrace turned to the torture of even more separation and isolation from the love I so badly needed.

Going to a Biomechanic

My wife had experienced some local and relatively mild back pain some time ago. She knew of a physician at a local university who called herself a biomechanic. Her office was many miles from my

home, and pain drilled through my pelvis at every bump in the
road.

Once in the biomechanic's office, I immediately detected the
domain of this woman's specialty. She approached me as if I were a
machine that had gone out of alignment. She lifted an arm here
and a leg there. She was much rougher than the plant lady who
knew of our oneness. I screamed in pain, and the biomechanic
said, "I know it hurts. You are all out of alignment. I'll manipulate
your muscles and bones to get you back in alignment, and you
should go home and try some exercises to get you back in shape
and straightened out."

"But I feel so sick," I said, "and the pain is unimaginable. It's like
I'm being eaten away down there. I know there is more going on."
Like the physiatrist, the biomechanic then attempted to use her
see-and-touch skills to journey across what psychiatrist Walter
Prince called the "enchanted boundary" that seems to separate the
mechanical world from the interpretive and spiritual world. [12]

"You have what I call the turtle syndrome," she said. "Due to all
your stress at this time of career change, you have pulled yourself
into your own body. See how bent you are? See how your head is
down there right inside your shoulder blades? Just like a turtle. You
must accept the fact of the closing of your clinic and come out of
your shell. You must work through this pain."

I went home and got even worse. I cried through the night, and
my wife called the biomechanic for help. The doctor wrote a pre-
scription for a slightly stronger painkiller, but no medication could
have worked. The pain was beyond the mechanical reach of medicines because my bones were being eaten away by as-yet-
undiscovered cancer cells.

On my last trip to the biomechanic, I could no longer walk from
the parking lot to the building. My wife had to find a wheelchair,
and for the first time in my life, I was wheeled through a crowded
waiting room. The doctor asked me to turn over on the exam table,
and I could not move. By now, still undiagnosed and unbeknownst
to me, I barely had any hips at all. My entire pelvis was crumbled,
leftover diseased bone and muscles torn away from where bone
used to be. I said that I was afraid that if I turned over, my leg
would fall off the table and the pain would be beyond description.

The biomechanic crossed her arms and said sternly, "Work
through the pain. You can do it." I struggled like a beached whale,

and my leg flopped off the table. I nearly passed out from the pain as muscle tore away from bone already dismantled by the cancer cells. I swore and cried as the biomechanic stood and watched.

"It's going to take a lot of work, and your impatience and anger won't help," she said. "Maybe you should try an acupuncturist. Your healing energy is blocked by your anger." Again, even as she spoke of energy, her metaphor was one of mechanical traffic jams.

One of the most destructive recent trends in so-called psycho-somatic medicine is the unsubstantiated claim of emotional cause of illness. What might have been a source of healing through hope, prayer, and a new view of cosmic rules as they apply to a person's own life has become, sadly, a new diagnostic system of patient blaming.

Going to a Quantum Healer

The next stop in my desperate quest for help was at the office of an acupuncturist. Needle after needle was placed throughout my entire body as the acupuncturist said, "It's not supposed to hurt. Why do the needles hurt you? I've never had a patient tell me that these little needles hurt. They're in the right chakras." He seemed unaware that, while he vehemently denied a mechanical approach to healing, he was viewing the acupuncture procedure through the cause-and-effect paradigm.

Using the language of the quantum realm of energy rearrange-ment, the acupuncturist said, "I can feel with my hands that the energy has all focused here in your back and hips. We'll move it down and out with several acupuncture treatments. You have a very severe sprain."

This specialist approached my case as if energy were a "thing" to be "moved." He was attempting to move electrons with hammers and nails. He spoke of energy, but he dealt only with particles. Like the biomechanic, this quantum healer failed to look for realms of reality other than his own. When my problem seemed unresponsive to their efforts, these specialists responded by trying even harder to apply their one realm of healing. Doing "more of the same" is something all of us do when confronted by a problem that confounds us, but this tendency is a key roadblock to making miracles, which calls for openness and unconventional thinking.

After several painful drives over a long distance to visit the acupuncturist, my last visit was the worst of all. "I'm not sure why it's not working," he said. Today, I'm going to use the most radical treatment I have." He stuck more than 100 tiny needles in my body and turned on an electrical instrument designed to send a small charge through my body. My muscles quivered, my hands and feet spasmed inward, and pain raged through me. I felt as if I had been electrocuted.

As I struggled out of his office, I had to be supported by my wife. It took almost fifteen minutes for me to "walk" 100 feet to our car. Hearing my groans and seeing my straining, the quantum theorist offered one more desperate word of advice. He said, "You are not reacting in the correct way. You look weaker than ever. Try soaking in epsom salts. That sometimes helps a sore back." I remember my mother telling me to do the same thing when I was a child and I became frightened that my doctors, without openly saying so, were now displaying their helplessness. I represented their failure, and I felt that they did not really want to see me again.

I never returned to the holist, the physiatrist, the biomechanic, or the acupuncturist. No one had helped, so I did what so many of my patients did. I entered the "plea-bargaining phase" of serious illness. After dozens of painful tests and treatments, I decided to forget the doctors, accept the punishment of living in terrible pain, and try to go on with my life. If only things would not get worse, I would try to accept the sentence of living in this misery.

The Spirit's Mistake

It was near Christmas of 1988, and I managed to struggle to my Maui home, hoping that the warm climate would help. With the support of my courageous family, each of whom were bruised, sore, cut, and callused from hoisting me from place to place, we tried one more time to "just go on living." I was saddened as I saw my family's bodies being wracked with pain because of my pain, and I realized how much a part of one another we really are.

As the Christmas decorations were hung, I sensed a preparation for mourning instead of celebration. The usual glee of our traditional family celebration was absent in spite of my wife's courageous efforts to carry on just as she had done during all of our family crises. I still didn't know it, but I was slowly dying. I sat on the beautiful Maui beach and watched my family and friends swimming. I loved to surf in the rolling waves. There seemed to be a symbolic parallel between trying to find a pattern in the roaring chaos of the waves to catch just the right spot to whisk you safely along and the challenges of transitional life problems. One of my Hawaiian neighbors called it Zen and the art of surfing. Now, I felt as if I were a child being punished by being made to sit on the beach and watch everyone else having fun and having life. I felt my tears warmed by the Maui's sun. My spirit dragged me limping to the water to try to swim in the warm and buoyant ocean.

As often happens in Maui waters, an unexpected wave several feet higher than the rest crashed toward me. I had thrilled to this safe emergency hundreds of times in the past, but I had forgotten my immobility and pain. I was caught and tumbled helplessly for what seemed like an eternity. I was slammed like driftwood against the hard sand, and I heard the crack as I broke my shoulder.

I knew from this terrible fall that I was totally out of coherence with living. I couldn't seem to find the crest of the wave, to fit in with it, to go with it. I couldn't find my place in the wave; I couldn't get with "the way it was." I made the dangerous mistake of flailing helplessly against the force of nature when the safe way would have been to curl myself inward and roll with the turbulence and turmoil. I knew that something beyond my broken shoulder and chronically painful hips was dreadfully wrong.

The pain of my broken shoulder was so much less than the pain caused by the cancer that I simply let the shoulder heal on its own. I had been let down by doctors so many times before that I felt that this type of injury would just have to heal alone. I know better now, but my judgment was clouded by my helplessness, pain, and the seductive "surrender secretions" of the neurochemistry of death that was circulating through me.

More Mechanical Misery

I flew back to Michigan to see yet another doctor. I seemed to be doing better because I was doing everything I could to adapt, but in fact I was getting worse. In hopes of a fresh approach and a different view of my pain, I went to a rheumatologist and board certified internist who injected medicine directly into my tumor as a treatment for what he said was an inflammation in the pelvic area. "You've really got a bad back there," he said. I went home, and the pain that I was sure could get no worse, worsened.

The Danger of Being *Too* Tough

Throughout this journey through the realms of reality, my family and I were *too* successful at survival. While I have pointed out that "spiritual toughness" is an important part of miracle making, overtraining to the point of spiritual numbness and failure to take necessary steps for diagnosis and healing is a very real hazard. We adapted too well and fought too hard. We had so often coped with crises and developed such a strong toughness response that pain was not having its necessary effect toward healing. In effect, we had become "spiritually muscle bound." We had dealt with the sudden death of our fathers, my wife's mother's stroke and sudden death, fertility problems, and the birth of two impaired children. We were tough, and our own coping skill prevented us from the panic that might have brought more immediate or sensitive help.

Because of the extraordinary support of my family, I was able to return in February 1989 to my home in Maui, where I managed to complete a book on *The Power of the Family*. I have since dedicated that work to my family for their saving of my life. It seems incredible that I completed a best-selling book while I was dying and suffering unimaginable pain. I am better able to see what happened to me now than when I was actually living through the tragedy. I will never know how I wrote that book through all of the pain, but on some level of reality, I suppose it was a way of reordering my life, a type of literary surfboarding.

My pain worsened and my walk deteriorated even further. I had several professional speaking engagements on my schedule, and I had never failed to honor a commitment to appear. I could only shuffle a few feet now, so my wife rented a wheelchair. I flew from one Hawaiian island to another by being hoisted in my wheelchair on and off planes with a forklift. I delivered my lectures about healing and miracles, but I stood in one place in such agony that tapes of these lectures show me grimacing throughout my talks.

While in Hawaii, and after my shoulder improved, I decided to try another doctor. I went to Honolulu to see an orthopedic physiatrist or a specialist in bone and muscle disease. He used a long, thick needle to inject me with steroids to ease the pain of my sore back. As it turned out, he was digging directly into my tumor and stimulating it to further growth. He, too, remained within his own realm. When I called him to report my worsening condition, he said, "Take some aspirin. Take three every five hours if you have to. Maybe you had better see some other specialist."

As I read through the book on family loving that I wrote in Maui during my suffering, I realize now that I knew I had cancer. I had even asked several of the doctors along the way, "Are you sure it's not cancer?" No one had listened to what I thought was wrong and why. No one thought that it was within my own reality that my illness was happening, not theirs. No one was alert to the fact that it was not against the rules to test a cancer and immune system researcher such as myself for the possibility of cancer of his own immune system. In retrospect, the clue of my book *Superimmunity* was a coincidence that should have been noticed. Instead of seeking the realms of reality where my disease was taking place, including the quantum energy realm where cell disruption first occurs and the interpretive realm where clues to the source of my pain were available (my first book, my lectures, my several earlier family crises), the realm of the see-and-touch reality was imposed on me. Just as I had struggled for my place in the chaos of that terrible wave in Maui, so my doctors and I had been unable to find the pattern, the crest or core of my crisis in the form of the energy disruption that was causing an overgrowth of cells.

Metaphors for Miracles

Miracles cannot be made if we do not look for a meaning in chaos or if we are frightened by the clutter and clamor of its force. If we try to correct chaos by squeezing it into one limited realm of reality, we cannot find the healing energy that helps us make our miracles.

In my case, metaphors for miracles were everywhere. Miracle markers to healing were evident in the "coincidence" of my first book on the immune system and cancer, in the "energy" sapped from me by the closing of my clinic and in the numerous family crises occurring so closely together, in my reports to my doctors that it felt "like something is eating away my hips," and in the deep conviction of those who loved me who so often said, "We know there is something terrible going on."

The doctors and I should have been *uncertain* and looked beyond the mechanical view of a "broken" or "strained" back. We should have seen that the *complementary* case was true: I *was* broken in that I was overgrowing. Cells were multiplying out of control. My disease was not to be found only on the local level of a break or strain or even a "lump." I also was suffering *nonlocally:* A system or waves of energy were disrupting my body. The Maui wave that threw me to the beach was telling us that my illness was caused by waves, not particles, but we were *observing* and looking only for particle pain. If there was any "break," it was in my *oneness* with my world because of my changing career and my struggle to find a new life. I was seeking new *realities* and trying to grow, but my body cells were outgrowing me! I can look back and see the metaphors for making miracles and the meaningful coincidences of my life, but I hope that you can use the six science secrets explored so far in the first seven chapters of this book with the remaining secrets of science discussed in the next four chapters to help you develop *foresight* rather than hindsight as your point of view for miracle making.

Calls for Help in the Night

At 3:00 and 4:00 A.M. Maui time, I would call various doctors in Detroit for help. "Take some aspirin," said one doctor. "Try to relax," said another. I tossed and turned in agony in what I had always thought was paradise, but even Maui seemed to fail me now. Instead of basking in the warmth and beauty of this secluded island, Maui now seemed to be a trap isolated from the "real" world where help might be. I know differently now, for the magic of Maui helped save my life.

I tried to shop for groceries, but in lifting one bag from the cart, I felt another ripping sensation in my hips. I screamed in pain, and shoppers in the store looked in amazement as an old woman helped me to my car. It felt as if a muscle had torn out part of the bone in my right hip. I would discover later that such destruction was exactly what was happening. I was literally falling apart.

I could no longer support my own weight. I was in constant

pain, and dying every day. I tried hot baths, cold baths, aspirin, meditation, screaming, crying, and swearing. I tried praying for help, but my prayers did not seem to be answered then. I know now that local time is not the best scale for measuring prayer response time. You read in chapter 6 about "the right kind of prayer," and I now know that prayer, in fact, helped save my life.

X Rays by Moonlight

On my last night in Maui, Maui helped me make a miracle. I lay on my bed watching the full moon over Haleakala Crater. The moon was so bright through the clear Hawaiian air that I could look down and see my body. Haleakala volcano was pointing to my illness. I saw a shadow across my hips, but there was nothing external to cast that shadow. Something within me did not allow me to dismiss this moonlight X ray—this coincidence of an object-less shadow. I knew something horrifying was wrong, and we went home to discover what the horror was. I wanted a bone scan or CAT scan that creates a computer image of my hips. I wanted to be checked for the terrible possibility of cancer.

The "coincidence" of the moonlight X ray pointed the way to my cure by casting a shadow on my hips. Subsequent tests designed to detect energy disruption in that area would show what the radiologists called a "massive shadow" in my hips.

My cries in the night had been answered by the moon illuminating the shadow of my illness. I helped make my miracle by *paying attention to the coincidence* of Maui's X ray. Something dark and deadly was in my pelvis. My family took me back to Michigan to be saved.

The Crisis Questions and the Realms of Reality

When I asked "Why me?" about my illness, the concept of differing realms told me that we all must experience all of the realms of living. We all must go through the joy and the pain, the happiness and sadness, the celebration and the grieving of the see-and-touch world just as we are protected and promised immortality by the divine existence of the many domains of reality. We are all suffering and healing on some level of reality all of the time. Chaos, not balance and order, is going on at some level of reality all of the time. Chaos is the natural state of things, and within the chaos lurks lessons for the making of miracles.

When I asked "Why now?" I realized that the concept of a "now" is a dimension of only one domain of reality; the see-and-touch domain that follows linear, local time. I could choose to see myself as being trapped by a "now" that was running out, or I could view my crisis as a challenge of transition through the timelessness suggested by relativity and quantum theory, which teach us that nothing is static and that *chaotic change is a form of evolving order.*

When I asked "Now what?" I learned that terrible pain and crisis was a call to see more in living than just a local life. It was an opportunity to move to a higher level of sanity. When the moon over Haleakala Crater shone on my pelvis in Maui, I felt sparked by the conviction that I was not just a lonely voyager on a sea of one cause and one effect. Some other energies, some other worlds, were moving alongside me.

When I asked "So what?" the impact of many realms of reality struck me with full force. Our miracles and our miseries alike are voyages of the human spirit through the realms of our divinity. When we are not limited by local laws or the necessity to solve problems only in the here and now, we are free to ride the waves of our spiritual energy through the adventures, both painful and joyful, of the development of the collective human soul.

Volcanoes, Lava, and Life

The last book I read prior to heading to my Michigan home for help was the book I mentioned earlier written by physicist Harold J. Morowitz titled *Cosmic Joy and Local Pain.* By coincidence, he too had visited Maui in his quest for a nonlocal view of reality.

According to Dr. Morowitz, "Chemistry alone is too limited for the full richness of the world. Wishing now to grasp ideas in a more global context than polymers and cells and tissue, I come to the geochemist's four spheres as a framework upon which to build an understanding."[13] He went on to suggest that the spheres of the lithosphere (earth), hydrosphere (water), atmosphere (air), and biosphere (the "fire" or energy of biological life) were metaphors for levels of understanding of our living, and he had come to Maui where these spheres seemed to merge clearly.

Here in Maui and as I write these words, I can see the Pacific Ocean, Haleakala volcano, the west Maui mountains, the islands of Linai and Kahoolawe, and the crescent-shaped top of an eroded volcano named Molokini. The trade winds are blowing strongly, and the crisp crackle of palm leaves fans the sweet smell of the several flowers.

I am sitting next to a protea plant gathered from the slope of Haleakala. It is a plant that gives off a life force so strong that it resembles an animal more than a flower, and it seems never to die. Four large rainbows are arranged along the slope of Haleakala. Every human sense is stimulated here, and every realm of reality—including each of Professor Mororwitz's spheres—is represented.

Morowitz suggests that the plate tectonics of the earth (the moving and shifting of the continents over the bedrock plates of the planet that created the volcanoes that I see outside my window in Maui) is a metaphor for the shifting influences on our development and our interaction with the cosmos. He sensed when he visited Maui that here is one place where the realities come to you with little effort on your part.

Even as I write these words, a volcano is spurting forth glowing lava on the Big Island of Hawaii. The lava burns and destroys as it rolls to the sea to be cooled and to create a new soil that soon will be covered with flourishing flowers and palm trees. Over my shoulder is the volcano Haleakala, older than the Kilauea volcano on the slope of Mauna Loa, Hawaii. Kilauea is still busy creating its island in the middle of the sea. As I pointed out earlier, if much of our world seems to be dying a little every day, the Hawaiian Islands are becoming a little more alive every day.

Lava from Kilauea recently destroyed an old Hawaiian town. One of the natives told me, "You know, brother, that we would sooner see lava over us than hotels. Lava will turn to life again. Hotels just bring us running people who use but never see our paradise. Lava is Pele's [the goddess of the volcano] pain. Hotels are man's mess and no life comes from them."

The terrible force and destruction of lava is symbolic of nature's way of infinite growing. I remember feeling as if there were burn-

ing lava in my hips and in my veins when I received my chemotherapy. The Latin root word for *lava—lavare*—means "to wash or
cleanse." For me, lava symbolizes that we are coming alive again
even as we cycle through the natural pain, death, rebirth, growth,
and flourishing of the life spirit. We are cleansed through chaos.

James Michener wrote, "Then one day, at the bottom of the deep
ocean, along a line running two thousand miles from northwest to
southeast, a rupture appeared in the basalt rock that formed the
ocean bed. Instantly, the rock exploded, sending aloft through the
19,000 feet of ocean that pressed down upon it columns of released
steam."[14] My "So what?" question is answered by the powerful, if
sometimes excruciating, eruptive energy of the chaos of change as
we move through the realities of our existence. From chaos, paradise emerges.

Metaphorically, the lithosphere may be seen as equivalent to the
see-and-touch world. The rocks, soil, and volcanoes respond to the
force of tectonics and the powerful gravity of their own existence.
The lithosphere is something we can touch. My illness and pain
were real and existed in a local world.

The hydrosphere—the oceans, lakes, and streams that are
pulled and pushed by the invisible force of the moon—is equivalent to the quantum world. Like quantum "stuff," water is pure
potential: It is ice, steam, and liquid all at once, and its form
depends on the observer and what conditions the observer chooses
to create. Similarly, my illness would become what I ultimately
made of it. My illness would become a diagnosis or a verdict,
depending again on what reality I created.

The atmosphere is equivalent to the cosmos: the world of the
very large going very fast. The air we need to breathe is densest at
sea level and becomes more rare as this layer of our life extends
outward. Our physical body is bound by its need for the air close
to earth, but our nonlocal spirit, which flies among the stars, has
no need for oxygen. My pain was local and thus attached to the
lower levels of the atmosphere, but my hope was spiritual and as
free as the energy of the quantum and cosmic domains. My pain
could never diminish my hope unless I allowed it to by ignoring
my capacity to make miracles. The local reality of pain does not
obliterate the nonlocal reality of the infinite spirit.

The biosphere is equivalent to the interpretive level of reality.

Our identity lives on this level, interacting with plants, water, air, and all of existence. My own healing would depend on my unity and harmony with all of the spheres of life and reality.

Finally, there is a fifth sphere around our earth. This is the "nosphere," or the thoughts, feelings, beliefs, and loving of all of us that radiate around us. We are a part of and surrounded by this nosphere, and it is equivalent to our spiritual realm of reality.

Ultimately, we create our own reality. We choose how open or closed we will be in our view of life. We choose what sphere or spheres we will travel in and in what domains we will allow ourselves to participate and learn. Prayer is the process through which we celebrate our oneness. Creativity is the process through which we move from realm to realm to make a reality that we can live well within.

As I sat in my airplane seat on takeoff from the Kahului Airport in Maui to return to the mainland for help, I knew that I would be back. I looked out my window as the plane banked and we headed out to sea. Again, I saw Haleakala Crater and the small dot of my house resting on its long and sloping hill. It was late afternoon and the sun was setting in its usual explosion of golden orange reflected on the fluffy clouds and filtered through the palm trees that seemed to be waving good-bye. The full moon had already risen over Haleakala, and a huge rainbow left over from the usual late afternoon clear and cleansing tropical showers arched from the very top of the volcano to end at what seemed to be exactly my Maui home.

I didn't know what was in store for me. I didn't know about the cancer, the chemotherapy, the surgery, the bone marrow transplant, and my near-death experiences that were all to come. Still, even through my fear and pain, I thought, "If I'm given the time, I know I'll be back." Then, as you will read in the next chapter, it occurred to me that "I'll have to make my own time."

NOTES

1. Lawrence LeShan and Henry Margenau, *Einstein's Space and Van Gogh's Sky: Physical Reality and Beyond* (New York: Macmillan, 1982).
2. *Ibid.*, 19
3. R. Cavendish, ed., *The Encyclopedia of the Unexplained: Magic, Occultism, and Parapsychology* (New York: Penguin Books, 1989), 167.

4. A technical explanation of how correlations are "stuff" in a quantum vacuum is presented in R. M. Wald, "Correlations and Causality in Quantum Field Theory," in *Quantum Concepts in Space and Time*, ed. R. Penrose and C. J. Isham (Oxford, UK: Oxford University Press, 1986).

5. David Finkelstein, "A Theory of the Vacuum," in *Philosophy of the Vacuum*, ed. S. Saunders (Oxford, UK: Oxford University Press, 1989), 1.

6. Tony Hey and Patrick Walters, *The Quantum Universe* (Cambridge, UK: Cambridge University Press, 1989), 130.

7. Baruch Spinoza, *The Philosphy of Spinoza*, intro. by Joseph Ratner (New York: Random House, 1927), 7.

8. Quoted in E. Cassirer, *The Philosophy of the Enligh:·nment* (Princeton, NJ: Princeton University Press, 1951), 41.

9. For a discussion of the significance and interpretation of miracles, one of the first and most famous explorations of this topic is found in David Hume, *Enquiry Concerning Human Understanding*, ed. L. A. S. Bigge (1758; reprint, New York: Greenword Press, 1980), chapter 10. For a current discussion of the issue of miracles, see Richard Swinburne, *The Concept of Miracle* (New York: Macmillan, 1970).

10. Reported in Newsweek, Oct. 22, 1990, 61.

11. For a description of the way in which laws of other realities are not, in fact, contradicted by paranormal events, see a letter written to (but unpublished in) *Science* magazine by Lawrence LeShan and Henry Margenau, *Einstein's Space and Van Gogh's Sky*, 256–257. They write, "It does not seem possible to find the scientific laws or principles violated by the existence of ESP."

12. The term *enchanted boundary* was coined by Walter F. Prince in *The Enchanted Boundary* (Boston: Boston Society for Psychical Research, 1930). The term is used to refer to an invisible but almost impenetrable wall between our "knowing" of the mechanical, see-and-touch world and our "knowing" of the other realms of reality (including the spiritual).

13. Harold J. Morowitz, *Cosmic Joy and Local Pain. Musings of a Mystic Scientist* (New York: Charles Scribner's Sons, 1987), 18.

14. James A. Michener, *Hawaii* (New York: Ballantine, 1959), 2.

8

SACRED AND PROFANE TIME

Making Magic Moments

Contrariwise, if it was so it might be; and if it were so, it would be; but as it isn't, it ain't.
> —TWEEDLEDEE, in *Through the Looking Glass*

If Today Was a Fish, I'd Throw It Back In.
> —FOLKSONG LYRIC

Maui's Heavenly Hook

I am sitting in the dark on my *lanai* in Maui. As I type these words, the only light is from the backlit screen of my portable computer. I notice a brighter light in the southern sky, and turn off my computer to look. It is the star constellation called Scorpius, named after its sweeping hook shape resembling a scorpion's tail, ending in a "stinger" of two major star clusters with more than five suns. The brightest star of the clusters, Antares, brightens the Hawaiian night enough to cast a glittering white path on the ocean.

Here in Polynesia, where the demi-god Maui dragged the Hawaiian Islands from the Pacific Ocean with a cosmic hook, Scorpius is called "the hook." Rather than the deadly stinging potential of a scorpion, the Polynesians see in this constellation a symbol of the dredging up of new life. This constellation is most visible in the first week in August, particularly on August 8, this evening when I am doing my final proofreading of this manuscript. The light I am seeing is nearly 500 million light-years old, and I am overwhelmed with the coincidence of the appearance of this stellar celebration of the completion of my book on the anniversary of the day I first became sick. I am humbled by my realization of the sacredness of the time we are given and stunned by our irreverence for the time we have.

In this chapter, I will describe the seventh secret of science: the fact that time is not linear and flowing. It is a function of whether we make time a sacred celebration of our existence or a profane process of passing through a series of fulfilled obligations.

The Backache That Was a Soccer Ball

My body was slipped slowly through a dark tunnel. X rays flew through me as I was inched click by click through the computerized axial tomography machine, or CAT scanner, designed to detect malformations inside the body. A dye that made my entire body flush with heat and my heartbeat quicken was dripping into my vein to provide a contrast medium. Suddenly, while I was still not quite in or fully out of the tunnel, the machine stopped.

I heard alarmed whispering at the console outside of the CAT scan room. A technician came in with tears in her eyes. I had worked at this hospital for years, and almost everyone seemed to know me. "Dr. Pearsall," she said awkwardly, "The doctor wants to stop the test here and ask you to wait outside."

The pain in my hips was still excruciating, even though I was now receiving pain medication injections. Three technicians helped me to get back into my wheelchair, covered me with several blankets, and draped one small blanket over my shoulders and head. I felt and looked like an old and dying man. The plastic shower cap they had placed on my head to prevent my hair from becoming caught on the machine made my scalp sweat, but I was too weak to lift my arm to take it off.

I was wheeled to my wife, who was waiting alone in the hall. Without looking at us, the technician said, "The doctor will be with you in a minute." We heard more whispering in the console room as other doctors rushed in to see the tracings of my hips. A hospital page called frantically for one of my doctors to report to the CAT scan room. Even though I was covered with blankets and still had warm dye dripping into me, I felt a terrible chill. The thick, chalky fluid I had been given to provide additional contrast medium for my intestines started partway back up from my stomach.

I could not move without pain. I held my wife's hand, and we tried in vain to cry. Things were so bad and so sad that tears seemed an understatement. We sat quietly, crying tearlessly. Time seemed to stop. The long, cold, tunnellike corridor that I had walked so quickly through when I used to visit my own patients was empty except for the echoes of the page calling for my doctor to report to the CAT scan room "stat."

Hospitals are in their own time zones. For a population of patients who are stripped of their clothes and placed in bed all day, there really is no regular night or day. There are only changing shifts and scheduled tests. We patients would lie waiting, worried, and afraid, for what seemed like hours outside a testing room while hospital workers and visitors rushed past in their own time zones. Now, my wife and I were experiencing the beginning of an entirely new sense of time that would come to be measured in sacred moments too often interrupted by profane periods of pain, fear, and suffering. Just as our clock had fallen from the wall when a doctor called with bad news, so our mechanical view of time had been shattered forever.

Finally, the radiologist approached us. She had been crying. "There's something terrible growing in your hips," she said. "We're taking a careful look, but it is growing all over. It has eaten away almost all of your hips."

I felt numb. I wanted to run. I wanted to disassociate myself from my body so that I would not vanish with it. I could not think, but responded in a childlike voice, "Is it terminal?" My wife pulled my shawl more snugly over my shoulders and head as the doctor laughed awkwardly, "Terminal? Well, what is terminal?" She laughed again nervously and said, "You'll have to talk to your own doctor." Then she walked quickly away.

In that one moment, my whole life had been declared over. In one quantum leap of seconds, I went from a life of pain and suffering to a direct confrontation with the end of my life. My doctor finally arrived. He stood over me and said, "I looked at the scan. It is very, very bad. It's a soccer-ball–size tumor. It wasn't a back sprain. It's cancer."

I will remember forever that deadly dyad of words. Words that change your life. I had felt the impact of a deadly dyad once before when I had arrived at the hospital too late to see my father alive. My brother and mother were holding each other, and my mother looked up. "He's dead," she said. Two words, and then total pain, helplessness, and a complete and sudden confrontation with the ultimate finality that characterizes our local existence. Now I heard "It's cancer," and I felt the same sting of despair.

My wife and I sat quietly and squeezed our hands tightly. "We'll have to start treatment right away," said the doctor. "But I won't lie to you. You only have a few weeks, maybe months. Of course, you never know. There are always miracles. But it looks very, very bad."

There Are Always Miracles

My CAT scan was completed and I struggled to dress to go home. My wife and I did not talk as we drove toward our house where my sons were eagerly waiting for the results of my test. My wife wiped tears from her eyes and said, "I'm sorry. Don't worry about my crying. We'll make it. I'm just still stunned, but we'll make it."

We drove in silence. I noticed all the trees that showed the slightest hint of buds. We passed the tree-lined paths in our neighborhood where we had walked and bicycled together, but these places now looked like old photographs from our family album. They were now the places where I used to be. They seemed lifeless.

I would have to wait through the weekend until a biopsy confirming my fate could be done on Monday. Hospitals stick rigidly to their time zone. Biopsies were not done on weekends and certainly not on the weekend of Easter Sunday, which this happened to be. I felt that my time, all time, had lost meaning. I felt that time literally had run out.

As we entered the house and our sons and dogs ran to us, I lost control of my bowels. The X-ray media and the deterioration of my hips combined to cause everything to drain from me. In front of my family, I messed in my pants.

I went to the bathroom to try to clean myself, but the pain caused me to fall in my own defecation. From here forward, my body would not be cared for by just me. The simple movements of cleaning and bending were agonizing.

My sons couldn't wait. They demanded to know what was wrong. I heard my wife tell my sons that "Dad has a tumor. It is cancer. It is very serious." I heard wailing cries, and I began to sob uncontrollably.

This most dramatic time in my life was happening, and I was not there with my family. As I tried in vain to clean myself, I became nauseated by the odor and panicked by the fact that I could not get up by myself. "Some psychologist I am. I'm busy lying in my own crap while my wife has to tell my sons that I am dying. By the time they see me, my whole world with them will have changed. My time with them will never be the same again."

The First Supper

Everything became quiet in our home. None of us knew what to say. Even our two dogs seemed confused and listless, and the pendulum on our grandfather clock in the hall had, for the first time since we bought it six years earlier, come to a complete stop. I shuffled urgently toward the clock, banging my walker on the ceramic floor one inch at a time. I had to get there. I struggled to open the glass door, but I could not see the handle clearly because of the tears flooding my eyes. I tried to support myself with one arm on my walker. It took almost all of my strength, but I managed to push the pendulum to start time again.

Family rituals go on, because they are the family's way of holding on to their own time against the profane march of local time. We would have our supper at our same time. We all sat looking at our food. My sons were trying to hide their tears. No one knew what to say. My wife spoke first. "We're going to celebrate Easter," she said through her tears. "We're going to go on. We're going to live now. We are not going to let this thing take away our lives. This is our first supper. We're going to make a miracle." We all cried together, and this time tears flowed easily and abundantly.

My wife and sons got up and came to me. They hugged me as the dogs jumped up to join us. We cried until there were no more tears left and then cried with dry eyes. I didn't know it then, but as you read in chapter 1, tears like these would help save my life in the intensive care unit by merging with my own tears to signal my existence in our local world. "This is our first supper in our miracle making," said my wife.

My older son, Roger, left the kitchen and walked the one-half acre to the river behind our house. He sat there alone until dusk. I wanted to join him, but I could not make it that far. His head was down and he just looked at the river flowing by. From time to time, he would toss a small stick into the stream and watch it float away.

The phone rang. It was someone calling me to complain that I had not called them back to confirm a lecture engagement. When I identified myself, the angry man said, "I am really upset with you. You have wasted my time. Why didn't you call when you said you would? I have a very busy schedule. There isn't enough time as it is, and this is a major crisis."

"I'm sorry," I answered. "I have a sudden health crisis of my own to deal with. I have to turn down your invitation for now. I've been busy with tests, and couldn't get back to you."

"Oh, no," he gasped. "This is the worst thing that could have happened. Thanks for nothing. Everyone really wanted to hear you. We looked forward to this for months, and now you have just wasted my time. This ruins everything." He slammed down the phone. I had had my first confrontation with the contrast between the profanity of our hurried local time and the sacredness of what the Buddhists call the Great Cosmic Time.

The Nature of Sacred and Profane Time

We tend to think about, measure, worry about, and watch time. For us in Western culture, time is real, linear, and the ultimate determinant of our life. Our almost universal impatience is a result of our being "time bound" and fearing that we will waste or run out of time.

As I waited for my biopsy scheduled for Monday, the weekend seemed to go by too fast and too slow. I was eager to have the biopsy performed so that at least I could know exactly what was killing me, but I needed much more time to contemplate what was happening to us. I thought of my life, my family, and the remarkable fact that, at this most terrible phase of my life and confronting my own death, I had realized that there did not seem to be a limit to my time after all. All I had, all I ever would have, and all that any of us have is "now."

We had our Easter Sunday dinner because my family claimed our own time from the grip of my disease. We were on our own "now" time: a time of merging moment by moment with everything that we can be conscious of. We exchanged small gifts and cards. As I opened a card from my wife, I began to cry again. "We're making a miracle now," said my wife as she hugged me. "Give us our time to make our miracle."

In our rush through profane time, we are always on our way out of the past and eagerly moving toward or anticipating the future. As a result, we miss our "nows" and, therefore, miss our lives. My confrontation with my mortality has cured me forever from missing the "nowness" of living.

Sensors and Censors: The Art of "Enlightened Denial"

The see-and-touch domain of reality was declaring me near death. On this level of reality, I would almost certainly die after some strong but usually futile attempts to kill the cancer cells that were killing me. There was no denying this reality.

On the other hand, the principle of oneness was holding me together emotionally and spiritually with my family; keeping me connected to our shared spiritual life and giving me the energy to keep going as I experienced the horrible fear that they might be losing me and that I could be losing all of them. We prayed that healing would take place and that God would work His will.

The principle of multiple realms of reality reassured me even through my fear and doubt. My disease would be real only in the way I chose to make it real. Like many people whose lives are threatened by serious illness, I developed an *enlightened denial*. On the see-and-touch level of reality, there was a mass of destruction in my body. To deny this level of reality would be to turn my back on the miracles of medicine that could help save my life. To function and feel *only* on this level of reality, however, would prevent me from mobilizing the energy from the other levels of reality. I could create the meaning of this crisis, decide how much energy this mass would have in my own life, and try to make the miracles to carry us through it. The doctors may have seen a "lump," but I knew from my work with my MM patients and from new science that my illness was as much an energy "jump" as a set of particles gone wild.

In his book *Vital Lies, Simple Truths,* author Daniel Goleman wrote, "Somewhere between the two poles—living a life of vital lies and speaking simple truths—there lies a skillful mean, a path to sanity and survival."[1] I suggest that this path is followed by *selective denial* of realms of reality in which we are at least temporarily powerless (as when we are diagnosed with a serious physical problem) and attention to realms in which we have the power to make our miracles (the power of the human spirit to alter events on the quantum level and thus affect the physical state). Enlightened denial is realm hopping to find a realm we can work in while denying realms that offer only hopelessness.

On the see-and-touch level of reality, we are physical *sensors,* but we are also *censors* in that we can select what we see and how we will interpret our world. Enlightened denial involves both processes: acknowledging the reality of a given situation and then denying that reality's stranglehold on our selection of coping strategies.

Similarly, the principle of observer participantcy teaches that we can "tell" time instead of allowing linear time to tell us what our reality will be. We give seconds and minutes their meaning. We do not live in "the" world; we live in "our" world. I would make up my own mind about the chaos of my cancer. Claiming my own version and value of time was a key step in my own miracle making because it freed me from a strictly mechanical criterion for happiness.

There Are No Time Limits

Yogis make themselves a part of time rather than allowing themselves to be ruled by time. If we learn the seventh secret of science—that time is relative and determined by our own ways of thinking about our lives—then we become a part of time instead of limited by it. Cancer forced this "personal relativity of time" on me. More and more every day, my disease drew my attention away from the dominance of a local, linear time toward a reverent merging with "now."

I waited on Tuesday for the results of my Monday biopsy. Now that I had "run out of time," I seemed to have more time than ever before. I began to see that the world was not made of simple beginnings and endings with predetermined measures in between. We are always in transition back and forth between the complementary aspects of our lives, not moving along a one-directional line between the stages of living.

My family and I began to see that one phone call about my condition did not have to move me further down the time line toward sure death. As we waited for the call about my biopsy, we began to feel the slightest hint of hope even at this darkest of times. This hope sprang from an evolving enlightened denial of an absolute time beginning with health and ending in disease and death. We were beginning to learn that chaos is a natural part of living.

Physician Larry Dossey writes, "This is the ultimate form of health—not the acquisition of an unblemished state of physical perfection, but the abolition of the opposites of health and disease, birth and death."[2] I had always done everything I could to avoid illness through exercise, diet, meditation, and an attempt to balance my life. The threat to my health now taught me that I had made a grievous error in thinking that illness was not a part of health and living. Illness and wellness together are part of the experience of the now in our living.

A New Meaning for "Now"

As I described in chapter 2, the glass clock that had been hanging from our wall for years fell to the floor just at the moment that the phone rang with the results of my biopsy and the doctor's announcement that my "time has probably run out." Quantum quakes from other levels of reality were breaking through to our awareness, causing the coincidence of our clock falling from the wall at just the "right" moment.

According to the laws of new science, our personal experience of time can be explained on both the quantum and cosmic levels. Cosmically, the speed of light (5,880,000,000 miles in one year) results in us seeing the light of a star "light-years" after that light was actually emitted. By the time we see the light of a star, that star's existence has changed. Thus when we admire Maui's hook in the sky over the southern Pacific, we are admiring a cosmic illusion. The cosmic now is a matter of how and how fast an observer is moving in his *own* space as he "sees" the speed of light.

Even the people we see are delayed and interpreted images of light, representing an existence of that person that is already history. Like the umpire in an earlier example of the observer participantcy principle, we are the umpires of our own games of life. The world itself is a cold, meaningless arrangement of particles and energy. When we see someone, our brains give meaning to the light patterns we receive. Light takes time to reach us and to be interpreted, so in this sense the person we are related to is already history! In terms of relative time, we are all cosmic illusions.

If we realm hop to the quantum level, we see, in the words of psychologist Dana Zahar, a "composite of already existing but ever fluctuating sub-selves—our selves as we were before 'now.' "[3] On the quantum level, we are ever-changing waves available for interpretation by people around us, who sense and censor what we will mean to them. "Now" is our local glimpse of a wave in progress: those brief moments when we pass from wave to particle and back to wave; from the sensation of "me" to "all of us and everything" back again to "me."

If we are trapped in profane time, we cannot perceive these "quantum time leaps." Miracle making is made more difficult because we are too busy looking back or forward to pay attention to the miracles available in the now.

Just as the sonic boom of a jet breaking the sound barrier can shake the clock off the wall, so the energy released by breaking our own personal time barrier to discover other realms of reality can knock the glass clock from our wall. Coincidences are the aftershocks of the breaking of the time barrier, whisking us at *transluminal speed* (transcending lumination, or the speed of light) to other realms of reality.

When something seems to "just happen" and to correspond meaningfully with what is going on in our life, the universal clock is making its presence known. Science cannot yet measure the breaking of the time barrier, but coincidences like the falling clocks and golden beetles I described in chapter 2 provide evidence that such transcendence has taken place. Coincidences are the clues to the passing of cosmic time.

Just a Miracle Moment

"Just for a moment, I was overwhelmed," said the mother. "The truck had not missed my little boy by more than inches. I should have run to my child, but I just stood there and relished the miracle of my son's being spared."

Most of us are aware of special, brief, beautiful, or frightening moments in our daily life. They may not be measurable by the reckonings of some atomic clock in a laboratory, but in coincidences we feel the miracle of our human spirit for just a moment. At such moments, time appears to stop. Everything seems to vibrate and condense into one coherent whole and we feel the rapture of an insight into the magnificence of our shared human soul.

Every coincidence I experienced and every synchronicity reported by my seventeen "miracle" patients seemed to last just for a moment. As soon as the moment is over, we feel drawn back to the local, see-and-touch reality of everyday life. Does the intensity of a "cosmic now" flash through our lives as a miracle moment?

Psychologist William James referred to the "specious present." The term *specious present* is used by psychologists today to refer to the span of time that our attention and awareness can allow us to experience as "now." Most laboratory research indicates that this "moment of now" lasts about twelve seconds. There are times when we seem to be briefly very aware of the beautiful and magnificent now. These are the "aha" times when we are intensely conscious of our living. Laboratory research indicates that our "aha's" and "oh no's" both have approximately a twelve-second psychophysiological impact.

By coincidence, new physics teaches us that the length of time it takes for the "coherence" of the Bose-Einstein condensate, mentioned in chapter 6, to occur (the sudden coming together of a system to be much more than the sum of its parts) roughly approximates that twelve-second "now" awareness. The "now" of a laser beam (one example of the coherence of a Bose-Einstein condensate) flashes for about twelve seconds. Our twelve-second "nows" in which we merge with the nonlocal world seem in this way to be connected to manifestations of "nowness" in the quantum and cosmic realms.

Think of the major moments in your own life. Remember how you reacted to very good or bad news. About how long did the initial reaction last? There is an initial flush of psychophysiological reflex, and everything after that is a reaction to our reaction. Just as the speed of the light of a star causes us to react to something that really does not exist in the local world, most of our psychological reactions are "to our reactions."

Quirks, Quarks, and Nobel Prizes

The 1990 Nobel Prize for Physics was shared by Jerome Friedman and Henry Kendall of the Massachusetts Institute of Technology and Richard Taylor of the Stanford Linear Accelerator Center. They won their prize for the discovery of the quark, the basic building block of all matter. The quark's existence is "implied" from the pattern of electrons ricocheting at large angles when they are hurled through a two-mile-long tunnel directly at a proton (a particle inside an atom). Instead of going through or around the proton, the electrons unexpectedly bounced off the quark, revealing a "something" that cannot yet be measured.

When scientists study the quark, their instruments reveal only the delayed effects of events caused by the quark's presence. Scientists are uncovering the miracle of this basic building block of the stuff of the cosmos by transcending the limits of their mechanical measures to come to know the essence of the quark on its own level of reality, using their imagination to realm hop to limitless discoveries. Researchers have won the Nobel Prize by going beyond the "quirks" of experiments to uncover the nature of the quark itself.

When people disappoint us, anger us, or behave in ways that seem to drive us away from them, they are presenting the quirks of their existence. When our relationships fail, they typically fail over the quirks of our humanness, not the basic building blocks or "quarks" of our essence as people. Dishonesty, infidelity, and other hurtful acts are the "light" emitted from the soul of a person and not the person himself or herself. If we learn to read beyond the delayed light that—like the electron paths around the quark—is only illusion of the true essence of the person, we can stop being light-years away from real loving and learning about our world.

People do not "make" us angry. We make ourselves angry at our angry reactions to our interactions with people. If we are miracle makers, we learn to transcend the speed of local time to interact with the true essence of a person rather than the image of that person. We do not react to our reactions—we interact with the real person through and in spite of the much-delayed image that strikes us on a local level. Miracle makers make the choice to *act* rather than *react* and to *merge with* rather than *look at* the events and people in their lives.

Star Struck with Cosmic Clout

"I have good news and bad news," said a doctor two days after I had been told that my time was running out. "The tissue sample showed that you have cancer, but you have lymphoma, which is a form of cancer that sometimes can be successfully treated. You have a form of lymphoma that has gone into your bones, but you do not have sarcoma (a usually fatal form of bone cancer). It looked like a sarcoma at first, but it isn't. We'll start chemotherapy right away."

The phrase "it looked at first like" is indicative of our tendency to react to images instead of essences, functioning too often as sensors rather than as censors, arriving at conclusions based on limited information. The light from a star is all we can "see," but if we contemplate the essence of a star and its gaseous, exploding essence radiating light through the cosmos to our eyes millions of years delayed from its actual cosmic bang, we experience stars on an entirely different level. We are no longer star struck by the illusion of a delayed light. Instead, we realm hop into the cosmic mysteries of the universe.

In about the twelve magic seconds that it took for me to hear and understand the doctor's good news, I went from almost certain death to referral for a treatment that might save my life. I now began to sense the essence of my illness and was less blinded by the frightening glare of its power.

I called everyone I knew to spread the good news. In my excitement, I temporarily forgot that I was now in for a chemotherapy treatment that my doctor called the "scorch the earth treatment." It was one of the most radical, intensive forms of chemotherapy. As my doctor pointed out, "If the treatment itself doesn't kill you, you have a good chance of surviving this thing."

"I'm not going to kill you with kindness," said my oncologist. "If we don't act aggressively, we may not succeed. Too often, doctors lower the chemotherapy dose because of the side effects, but the chemotherapy just can't do the job at those lower doses. I'm giving you the full dose. We'll go for a cure."

Going Beyond a "Deadline"

In a matter of days, I had gone from pain to death to hope to fear and now back to hope again. I experienced this time of my life as a series of moments, of immeasurable "quantum leaps." As I sit here in Maui writing, I notice that it is almost exactly two years ago that I first experienced pain in my lower back. I'm cured of my disease, and I also am free of the profane-time disease that so often robs us of the miracle moments in our lives. The "now" of my life has become my personal time. The falling clock in my kitchen had been a sign that the mechanical ticking away of my life would be replaced by a new awareness of the value of now.

Now, I feel every trade wind breeze and am up to watch every sunrise over Haleakala. I walk with my wife in every golden sunset, and I put my effort into knowing the sacredness of "now" rather than in preparing for the illusion of "later." I enjoy every moment as I write these words and watch the symbols appear from energy within me, to be stored on disks as energy imprints and to reappear as symbols every time I turn on my computer. These magnetic energy images appear like the musical notes on a score of music, but like a musical composition, together they constitute much more than a collection of symbols. The symbol particles merge into a unique wave of energy that transcends local time to have an infinite life of its own. I too have gone beyond the profane quirks of linear living to the sacred time of just being alive.

I feel free now of the profane pressure of what we so accurately call "deadlines." Traffic jams have become pauses for a chance to think. Busy signals are signs that I am still alive to be inconvenienced and to be busy. I have a new sympathy for broken things, because I know that the sacred laws of science explain that things, plants, animals, and I all share moments of breakage and rebirth on several levels. Coincidences are my clear reminders of the sacred time by which the laws of science work their magic. All lines are "dead" if they are viewed as mechanical minutes elapsing through endless obligations to meaningless ends.

The Myth of a Lifeline

My wife has purchased and rehung a clock on the wall of our kitchen. By doing so, she is counting on another principle of new science that stretches our common sense to the limit. Irish physicist John Steward Bell, founder of the theorem of simultaneity of events and the fact that *time does not flow in only one direction*, proved that two things can happen at exactly the same time even if they are a universe apart. He proved that although things seem on a local level to be happening in a one-way, cause-and-effect direction, on other levels of reality, there is no such linearity. Hundreds of experiments and mathematical equations now prove that superluminal or faster-than-light speed is possible, and objects on the other side of the earth from one another can change together at exactly the same time.[4] By rehanging a new clock, my wife has symbolically acknowledged that our time did not and does not "run" out, because there is no lifeline that is running.

Scientists know that light, like everything else, is both particle and wave. The superluminal particles that constitute these waves are called tachyons. Like the tiny water particles that reflect light to make a rainbow, they are not visible to the naked eye. When we see a rainbow, we do not say "Look at that wonderful pile of particles!" We are awed by the light wave of magic and beauty that looks like a rainbow. Once the particles rearrange themselves, however, the rainbow is "gone." It will, of course, come back again somewhere, sometime. Rainbows don't have lifelines; like us, rainbows are forever and timeless.

The scientific proof of the existence of superluminal, or faster-than-light, particles called tachyons explains the *possibility of retro-*

active causation or of *our present affecting our past.* Tachyons are examples of the quantum principle that it is an absurdity to fix particles and waves (quantum stuff) in time and space. Quantum stuff is potentially everywhere and exists "at all times." When tachyons go faster than the speed of light (the c in Einstein's $e = mc^2$) they explain the possibility of the present changing the past, just as linear concept of local time explains how the present can affect our future.

One-Way Signs in an Every-Way World

The possibility of actually altering the past is one of the most difficult scientific secrets to accept. We think that time is absolute, but in fact it is relative. Albert Einstein's theory of relativity helps us begin to understand that time is not fixed in a one-way system; that time is a matter of the timekeeper and not the clock.

To learn that time goes forward and backward, consider the classic statement made by Einstein that he often used to explain the relativity of time. He said, "When you sit with a pretty girl, two hours seems like one minute. When you sit on a hot stove for two minutes, it can seem like two hours. Now that's relativity![5] Time is relative to how we choose to think about and remember the events of our life. Psychologists have shown that things we think of as being bad seem to last longer than things we think of as being good. Thus how we choose to construct our past in our memories does, on some level of reality, alter that past!

What we see as a sunset is also the beginning of a sunrise. In space, there is no up or down because the local law of gravity is transcended. Our cosmos is not a one-way, one-realm system, and our time is free from these same limitations, opening the way to explain retroactive causation, precognition, and other psi or psychic phenomenon. Science provides many proofs that time is not one directional.

The Importance of Crying Over Spilled Milk

Physicist Roger Penrose, whose work I referred to in chapter 1, writes, "The deterministic equations of classical physics . . . have no preference for evolving in the future direction. They can be used equally well to evolve into the past. The future determines the past in just the same way the past determines the future."[6] The molecules of a puddle of spilled milk can reassemble themselves, flow back into a glass crackled back together, and the glass can fall back up to the table from which it fell. Spilled milk can unspill! Newton's laws and all of the laws of physics predict that such an event can take place.[7] Penrose writes, "Such coordination [coincidence] could occur only by the most amazing fluke—of a kind that would be referred to as 'magic' [a miracle] if it did occur."[8]

I believe that such coincidences and miracles *do* occur. I experienced such a miracle. We should "cry" and give great significance to the "spilled milk" in our lives because such spills are *not* irreversible events. The spills of our life are the chaos from which we are challenged to find meaning. In "the past," my hips were almost completely eaten away by cancer. "Now" my hips are completely intact and reassembled after their cells were "spilled." My family helped me make the miracle of undoing my past by not allowing me to surrender to local time, helping me to cry and hope over my spilled milk, and helping me to resist verdicts from modern medicine that told me that my time had run out. My family helped me expose the myth of absolute time, find the miracle of time's relativity, and resist the constant temptation to surrender to the time limits imposed on me.

As I pointed out, Bell's Theorem proves that particles a universe away can change together at exactly the same moment. In other words, these particles can experience simultaneous changes of their lives back and forth through time in any direction. Modern physics thus proves that a cause can be an effect.[9] In Wheeler's two-slit experiment described in chapter 7, photons experienced a different past (being a wave or particle) depending on what happened to them "later" as they went through the slits in the wall and depending on what we asked or expected from them in our "now." In the quantum world, electrons can make a transition from a higher energy state (faster spinning and motion through orbits) to a lower energy state (slower spinning and remaining in a given orbit) and back again in what is called the "quantum U." There are no one-way signs in the quantum world.

Just as doctors view "impossible" cures as "quirks of spontaneous remission," many scientists view the faultless mathematical proof of simultaneity and retroactive causation as a "quirk" of science. I view such findings as the cornerstones of an uncommon consciousness that can accommodate the existence of many realms of reality and the relative, directionless nature of time.

Ritual as Time Travel

One reason why ritual is so important in our lives is that through ritual we bring the past to the present, reconfirming our oneness with the past and the relationship of the present to the past. Rituals allow us to experience the relativity of time. Our most significant rituals seem to operate independently of time. Christmas traditions, removing the Torah from the Ark, and singing "Happy Birthday" are all rituals that help us reexperience what has already happened. They celebrate the constancy of the human spirit and the power of belief, and they bring the history of our shared being into the now. We are sometimes overwhelmed by emotion during our rituals in part because we actually experience the past as a real part of now. Even certain smells and sounds can trigger a flood of sensation and emotion that catapults our past into our present and our present back to the past. The power of ritual rests in its ability to merge present and past into a profound "now."

Through our rituals, we are given the opportunity to feel both the agony and joy of our past and present. When Charles Dickens's Ebenezer Scrooge was guided through his life by the spirits of time, he finally said what all miracle makers say: "It's not too late. I can do it! These are not the signs of the way things have to be." Our rituals help us remember that it is never too late to make miracles, to learn to celebrate the glory of our existence and to correct and redirect the energy in our own past.

Miracles are available to us when we realize that peace can be made with a deceased relative with whom we argued our lives away. We *can* "take back" our angry words and even say "I'm sorry" and "I love you" now and know that our words have an impact on our pasts. Any change can have an effect on any thing at any time.

We do not have to spend our time trying to "read" the future and mourn the past. We can get busy changing some of our pasts. Our pasts, as well as our futures, are ours for the making if we free ourselves from linear time. For Ebenezer Scrooge and for all of us, it's never too late, because *late* is a concept that has meaning only in the linear realm of reality.

Ritual is one way of "personalizing" time. My family made sure that every one of our rituals remained intact during my illness and treatment.

"We'll drag you to Christmas Eve dinner if we have to," said my wife. When I had broken my shoulder in the waves off the Kamaole Beach in Maui, my family took turns lifting my arm so that I could eat Christmas dinner. Our family rituals kept me in the "now," free from terror and the tyranny of the future. Doing this actually helped to alter a past assigned to me through medical verdicts that could have predetermined my present and future. My "medical history" was altered in my favor. Of my cure, my oncologist said, "It's a miracle. It's as if this disease never happened." On some levels of reality, he is exactly right.

Attending My Own Funeral

Another coincidence of time happened to me just before I began my chemotherapy treatments. I was scheduled to lecture to a large church audience. They had to lift me on stage in my wheelchair. I sat alone facing the large, silent congregation that had expected to see me as my usual energetic and highly mobile self. The organist played a song before my talk. The song was from the play *Fiddler on the Roof*, and it is called "Sunrise, Sunset." I felt that I was attending my own funeral.

The coincidence of my hearing, in a church, this song of life's rhythm, on the eve of my struggle for survival, just before a lecture on the making of miracles, was so piercing that I could not stop my eyes from flooding with tears. I didn't want to cry in front of this large group, but my wife sitting in the front row saw my tears. She smiled, held her thumb up in the air, and moved her hand in a circular motion of a number eight for the eight letters in "I love you." I could see from my angle that this number eight was also the symbol for infinity. It was the sign of the sacredness of time, and I merged with the "now" of the moment instead of my fear of the future. I could go on with my lecture, using it as a ritual reaffirmation of the possibility of miracles.

Exactly one year later, to the day, I returned to that church to lecture again. When I was introduced, I strode in and hopped up onto the stage. As I started to speak, the audience rose in a long, tearful standing ovation. I cried with them as I realized how relative time was. I had been to death's door and back, yet it felt that I had never left this state. I was awed by the irrelevance of clock time and the power of a sacred, relative, personal time.

Setting your own "time limits" by deciding how you will reconcile past, present, and future is central to the quality of your life. If we throw a pinch of salt over our shoulders when we knock over the saltshaker, we reveal a ritual based on "superstition" (i.e., acting in the present to avoid negative future consequences). If we put the salt back in the shaker, we reveal a "retrostition," or the idea that we can "put the past right." If we allow our lives to be governed by our need for "retrobution," or the attempt to avenge or correct a past insult or injury, we are trapped in a painful past of anger and hurt. If we brush the spilled salt aside without a thought, we live a local and somewhat reckless life of the here and now. We must choose how we will interpret the chaos of our world and what meaning we will give to the events in our lives. If we say that "something" makes us angry or happy, we are surrendering to a cause-and-effect view of the world. When we say, "I make myself happy or sad," we empower ourselves to live in a world of our own making.

Impossible Events Do Not Happen

We make meaningful miracles by accepting the impossible-sounding fact that everything is possible at any time. Scientific experiments show that "impossible" things cannot happen, but *the possible things that do happen are miraculous.* Several such studies are cited by authors John and Brenda Denner.[10] The Denners describe several studies of cosmic time principles. Most intriguing is their review of what are called "remote perception" experiments.

In these remote perception studies, a "sender" (a person who has never met the receiver) is told to transmit a message to a "receiver" who is up to 6,000 miles away. Through computer analysis, the accuracy and frequency of the receipt of these psychic messages through time are scored. Statistically significant success in sending messages in this way has been achieved and verified in dozens of other experiments.

Remarkably, the receiver in these "time travel" experiments often "gets" the message from the "sender" as many as three days *before* the message is actually sent! Several experiments (some conducted by our government in the effort to train psychic spies to match those already practicing their uncommon vision in the USSR) have proven the possibility of remote viewing.[11]

A New York artist by the name of Ingo Swann and his friend Harold Sherman could report accurate observations of the weather conditions on Jupiter, Mars, and Mercury that were confirmed *years later* by National Space and Aeronautics Administration (NASA) satellite missions.[12]

I hope you will use my personal experiences and the new science principles described here to explore how the realms of reality mingle and influence the times of your life.

The Birds and the Bees

One recent coincidence providing evidence of the role of sacred time in my own life occurred on my recent return to Maui to write this book. As we entered our home, we paused to savor the moment of our return to our peaceful, healing place. Instead of the usual hush, we heard a loud buzzing mixed with what sounded like hundreds of birds chirping.

"The birds and the bees are greeting us," said my wife. "They're singing a song of our renewal and rebirth." She laughed. Even though she was partly joking, my wife and I shared what seemed like about twelve seconds of a special sacredness, appreciating a meaningful synchronicity of nature that symbolized the miracle of my living, the buzzing of cells being reproduced by my healthy bone marrow, and the Bose-Einstein condensate of the wonderful oneness created from the spontaneous coming together of each individual bird and bee.

Later, we discovered that hundreds of bees had built a nest in our air-conditioner and that a family of birds unique to Maui, yellow-green amakihi birds, had built a nest on the top of the air-conditioner. The buzzing and singing would have been an annoyance before I learned the lessons of oneness, relative time, and the miracle of meaning within the apparent chaos of life. Now that I knew these secrets of science these sounds were a triumphant welcoming song in celebration of our return to my healing place.

The chemotherapy had been pure torture. Burning chemicals had stung my veins until it was almost impossible to find a place to insert the needles. Nausea, diarrhea, and painful mouth sores kept me awake through the night. Drinking glasses of baking soda mixed with warm water to prevent the acidic effects of the chemotherapy from burning away my bladder required several retchings before I could keep the liquid down. The support of my family seemed to provide an energy more powerful than the toxic treatments, and that carried me through the torture. The knowledge that I was never alone or separate from my loved ones and my constant rediscovery of our power to influence what was happening through our observer participantcy allowed me to withstand the awesome power of the chaos without surrendering to the panic and fear that were always with me.

Despite the powerful oneness I felt from my family's loving, there occurred moments during which I did feel an almost complete panic. As unpredictably and suddenly as the meaningful coincidences occurred in my life, just as suddenly I would feel overwhelmed, frightened, angry, and helpless. I would begin to sob without warning. I would bang my hands on the bed in desperation and I resented everyone who was healthy and able to walk. My wife came to call these times my "mess moments."

Miracles Aren't Always Nice

Following my first phase of chemotherapy, I had begun to walk again. Thanks to my family and in part to my dog Hana who insisted on my effort and practice, I took first one step, then three. I remember the look on my wife's face when I first walked into the kitchen without my walker.

"Well, a magical moment!" she exclaimed and held me. "God knows, I've had to put up with a lot of your mess moments."

We often see only "positive signs" as miracles, but the principle of complementarity stresses the dualistic nature of life. *All coincidences have meaning.* The gorgeous bougainvillaea plant around my home in Maui has terrible thorns, and every time I prick myself on the barbs within the beauty, I remember that the same cosmic joy that makes this wonderful plant also is causing me my local pain.

Having gone through my own best and worst of times, I am

convinced that there is an order in our living, and like the matter and antimatter of the quantum world, for every magic moment of insight and celebration, there are "antimoments" of pain and fear. As little Patsy warned, we must be able to wait for "how it is" and pray for "Thy will" to be done rather than panic during our moments of suffering.

Particularly at those times of "mess moments," we must just "be" rather than "do"; we must choose equanimity over panic and come to see the messes as a normal and necessary part of the natural chaos of illness and healing.

Let the Bad Times Roll

Every one of the seventeen miracle patients that I studied reported that there were moments of misery that paradoxically generated an energy and alertness that motivated further healing. Unless the "mess moments" were interpreted as the ticking of a linear clock and slow but sure movement toward ultimate failure, the times of suffering were stimuli toward a new commitment to make miracles.

"It's remarkable how, when I would feel a little better, the bad times seemed to be a part of bringing on the good times," said one of the seventeen miracle makers. "I guess you can't tell time by just marking the good times or you wouldn't have all the time you have. You'd always be at half time."

This man, who eventually overcame a sarcoma that doctors said would kill him in months, was referring to a more sacred view of time than "just letting the good times roll." We have to accept that the bad times roll too, inextricably enfolded with the good.

Another Fine Mess

The chemotherapy had been a remarkable success. The pain was greatly reduced and I was walking again. To assess the success of my treatments, my oncologist scheduled a bone marrow test and another CAT scan. As I described earlier, no one could believe that my X rays were my own. My hips had grown back. The cancer was completely gone.

When the doctor came in to do my bone marrow test, he seemed unusually quiet, but proceeded to work. The process of having bone marrow removed is similar to what a plant must feel when it is suddenly pulled up, roots and all. Nurses had to hold me down as the needle burrowed through skin, muscle, and bone to the very core of where my physical body is reborn every moment of my life. The pain of the suction when the marrow was withdrawn almost caused me to lose consciousness.

As I rested after the procedure, I asked my doctor if he had seen the results of my CAT scan. He said that he had, and then asked that my wife be brought in. I knew what that must mean. Something was terribly wrong.

"It's a miracle, all right," said the doctor. "The cancer in the bones is gone and you have completely new hips that have regenerated like magic. You're walking again. Unfortunately, something now is showing up in your abdomen. It might be scar tissue, but it might be something else. We'll have to check it out."

"Moments," I thought. "Moments. From a miracle to a mess in a moment." It seemed a fast twelve seconds of transition from elation back to fear.

A gallium scan was done by injecting a radioisotope into my vein, or what was left of my vein. I stood for several minutes in front of a large, silent machine that scanned my entire body for scintillations of energy where there should be no such scintillations.

"Everything looks fine," said the technician. "Just wait until the radiologist checks it over, and then you can go. Everything we saw on your earlier CAT scan is gone, and the gallium scan looks good. Congratulations." The technician is not supposed to give so much information or be trained to interpret tests, but many technicians have seen far more X rays than the doctors have and they've learned to spot trouble. This technician was someone I knew, and she wanted to help cheer me up.

We sat for what seemed like hours. Relatively speaking, bad news travels slowly. A hospital page went out for my doctor and other doctors, and they hurried into the X-ray reading room. "A mess moment," I thought. "Another damned mess moment." I kept telling myself that things would balance out. No matter what was wrong, something also could go right.

"Well, we have another fine mess. I'm afraid there's another tumor in there," said the doctor. "We'll have to do exploratory abdominal surgery to see exactly what it is."

Don't Just Do Something; Sit There

The surgeon said, "Abdominal surgery is no walk in the park. The preparation is lousy. You have to drink almost a gallon of terrible-tasting stuff, and then you'll crap all day. Then you'll have gas and a tube put down your throat into your stomach. I'm so sorry, but I'll do my best to make it as tolerable as possible."

My surgery revealed that I did not have a return of my former cancer. Instead, I had a *different* form of cancer.

"Can you believe it?" said my doctor. "Two for the price of one. It's like you're a surfer trying to ride the waves. Up and down, up and down. Just don't wipe out on me now."

I wondered if this doctor knew about my home in Maui and my love of surfing. I did feel as if I had been wiped out by a massive swell of waves. I was weak and sick from the surgery and I was vomiting every fifteen minutes, so I could not focus clearly on the challenge that lay ahead.

The Indolence of Waiting

Once I recovered a little strength, my wife and I waited again in the doctor's office to discuss my case. It seemed as if we had spent our life together sitting in offices waiting for someone to give us bad news. We had waited to find out that we would never be able to have children, only to discover that we could. We had waited to be told that our new baby had cerebral palsy and would never walk, only to find out that in spite of his handicap, he would walk and flourish. We had waited to be told by teachers that our other son might never talk or attend school, only to find out that he would graduate from high school and go on to meet the challenges facing every young adult. We had waited together to find out the results of a mammography for a very suspicious lump in my wife's breast, only to find that the lump was a harmless cyst. Now, we waited again.

"I'm afraid it's an indolent tumor—a very slow-growing tumor.

This type of cancer is not treatable," he said. "You could be dead in months." In the twelve seconds of a "specious present" that it takes for shocking information to set in, everything seemed to be over once again.

"Of course," he added, "There is the possibility of a bone marrow transplant. It's a very risky procedure, but there is some new evidence that it may actually cure indolent tumors. It's still experimental, but it is at least worth looking into. We'll refer you to the BMT, or bone marrow transplant, center. Your own marrow is clean, so you might qualify for an autologous bone marrow transplant. They'll take out your own marrow, give you whole-body radiation and extensive chemotherapy to kill the tumor and any remnants of your first cancer, and then put your stored marrow back in and hope that it comes back to life. The radiation and chemotherapy will kill the bone marrow left in you, because it kills anything that is growing, including your immune system. When they put your stored marrow back in, they pray that it regenerates itself so it can produce your blood cells. It could be a cure if it works, but as many as half of the patients who get these transplants don't make it."

We were off again to yet another office to wait together for yet another verdict on my life. To get through this mess moment, I used the seventh secret of science—the sacredness and relativity of time—to answer yet again the four crisis questions.

The Four Crisis Questions and the Time of Our Life

When I asked "Why me?" during my diagnosis and treatment, I looked to the principle of retroactive causality and simultaneity. If I saw my suffering as "just me," then I became a blip on a finite time line that would ultimately end in meaningless oblivion. If I saw my illness as relative and reactive to my own sense of time, I was free from the pressure to get better quickly. I also had the larger vision of seeing my life as a coherent whole of past, present, and future. My healing energy then was free to go in all directions at once. I could look back on my life for meaning, direction, and for the rituals that would bring the fond memories of my past to help me heal in the present. I could tune intensely in to every moment I had now to embrace and love my life with my family. I could contemplate the implications of my future because I knew we would make a miracle. Healing is not a "getting ready for the future" thing; it is a process of timeless faith in the perpetual human spirit.

When I asked myself "Why now?" during my several mess moments, I was forced to realize that there is only now. I may be able to understand and experience "now" only in brief quantum spurts through the clues of coincidence and sychronicities, but the worse the crisis, the more I seemed to experience "now." As soon as I learned that *time did not have to run me* and that *time did not have to make me run*, I was able to understand that *no one's cosmic time ever runs out*.

When I asked myself "Now what?" I realized that I was allowing myself to be pressured by a linear sense of time to do something that would help me "manage" the time I had "left." Once I learned that time is not a concrete entity, I knew that no one can "manage" their time. All we can do is experience our life to the fullest not by trying to save or keep time but by realizing that now is all the time we have. We don't have to wait for time to "pass," because we make our own time. When we make our own time, we have all the time in the world.

One reason why people who are given a second chance at life typically choose to "spend" their time fishing, sitting, talking, and thinking rather than running around the world trying to "do it all" is that by trying to "be" instead of "do," we can feel much more alive in the "now." When we celebrate every moment we are living in sacred time.

When I asked myself "So what?" the seventh science secret taught me yet another important choice in the making of miracles. If we do not actively and consciously choose the time we will keep, then we will be kept by time. How rushed we feel, how burdened we are with getting things and getting things done is a function of our decisions about time. The answer to "So what?" is that we can choose the pace of our living. It is "why" we go at a given pace that matters, not how fast we go. In my own case, rushing to make more money to get more things results in a profane time of obligations and pressure. Rushing to write and lecture about miracles that may help thousands of people results in a sacred time of oneness.

The Choice of Our Lifetime

Think about your daily life. How do you choose to "spend" your time? Author Jorge Luis Borges wrote, "You can't measure time in days the way you can money in dollars because every day is different." Every moment is different and dependent on how we choose to see that moment.

To discover your choice of time, take just one sample recent day and try to re-create it in writing, right down to the hour or minute. Now, record your idea of a miracle day. Hour by hour, how would you ideally be spending your time? Is there a close match between the "real" days and the "dream days"? The more different these two days are, the more likely you are to be missing the opportunity to make your own miracles.

Taking Your Time Pulse

I also suggest that you take your "time pulse." I have done this assignment with hundreds of patients, and it is one of the easiest ways of determining the time someone is marching by.

Sit down someplace quiet where you can see a clock with a second hand. Wait until the second hand reaches the top, and then close your eyes. Try to guess exactly when one minute is up, and then open your eyes. If you are really running on profane time, you may need someone to help you with this technique because you may be so rushed that you give up before the exercise is complete! When I asked one busy business executive to try the time pulse exercise, he said, "I will sometime. I don't have the time now."

Were you short on your estimate? Most people are. Some of my patients called time at less than fifteen seconds! All of my seventeen miracle patients, however, were long on their estimate. I had one patient who had almost died twice. She called time at more than five minutes. "I'm sorry," she said. "I just can't tell this type of time anymore, and I don't care."

The longer your estimate, the more close you may be to running on sacred time. The further you fell short of the minute, the more attention you should be paying to the sacred time of pausing, thinking, and just "sitting down and shutting up."

The eighth sacred secret of science, the rule of forceful fields discussed in the next chapter, also influences our sense of time. If you feel that you are a part of and constantly being revitalized by force fields around you, you may not allow what one of my patients called "local daylight ravings time" to dictate your life.

NOTES

1. Daniel Goleman, *Vital Lies, Simple Truths: The Psychology of Self-Deception* (New York: Simon & Schuster, 1985), 251. In this book, Goleman suggests that "selective attention" can offer us relief at times of suffering because such denial is a form of "psychic analgesic." He feels that denial can inhibit the stress response and reduce the flood of stress chemicals that can interfere with healing at those times when more healing chemicals and painkillers (the endorphins) are needed.

2. Larry Dossey, *Recovering the Soul* (New York: Bantam Books, 1989), 240.

3. Dana Zohar, *The Quantum Self: Human Nature and Consciousness Defined by the New Physics* (New York: William Morrow, 1990), 120.

4. For a clear description of Bell's Theorem and its proof and applicability in everyday life, see Nick Herbert, *Quantum Reality* (New York: Anchor Books, 1987).

5. Psychologist Robert Ornstein has researched the "psychology of time." He has shown that the fewer the number of events in a given mechanical unit of time, the shorter it will seem; and the more that is remembered in a given situation, the longer it seems. Ultimately, our sense of time is constructed out of our memories of experiences. Your past is actually psychologically changed by how you choose to remember it! See Robert Ornstein, *On the Experience of Time* (London: Penguin Books, 1969). Other research has proven that people perceive and remember an interval containing a successful event as shorter than one with a failure. We "make our time" independently of clock time. See J. J. Harton, "An Investigation on the Influence of Success and Failure on the Estimation of Time," *Journal of General Psychology* 21 (1938): 51–62.

6. Roger Penrose, *The Emperor's New Mind* (New York: Oxford University Press, 1989), 306.

7. *Ibid.*, 306.

8. *Ibid.*, 306.

9. J. A. Wheeler, "Genesis and Observorship," in *Foundational Problems in the Special Sciences*, ed. R. E. Butts and K. J. Hintikka (New York: Reidel, 1977).

10. John and Brenda J. Denner, *Margins of Reality* (New York: Harcourt Brace Jovanovich, 1987).

11. Several experiments have been conducted with persons detecting computer assigned locations by psychic ability. See R. Targ and K. Harary, *The Mind Race: Understanding and Using Psychic Abilities* (New York: Ballantine Books, 1984).

12. For a description of several studies such as the remote vision studies and secret government work on the efforts by the USSR and the United States to engage in "psychic spying," see R. Targ and H. Puthoof, *Mind Reach: Scientists Look at Psychic Ability* (New York: Dell, 1977).

9

VITAL VIBRATIONS

Learning That Life *Is* Fair

> Technological progress is like an axe in the hands of a pathological criminal.
>
> —ALBERT EINSTEIN

> Technology is a way of organizing the universe so that man doesn't have to experience it.
>
> —MAX FRISCH

Playing Fair with Life

When I would groan and cry in pain, it would seem to me that I was being punished unfairly. I constantly asked the four crisis questions of why me, why now, now what, and so what. As I squirmed and searched for any position that would at least diminish the throbbing pain, I would weep, bite my blanket, hit my fists on my pillow, and scream "It isn't fair!" Every nurse and doctor answered me the same way: "Life just isn't fair."

We were all wrong. Life is not unfair. We are unfair in our expectations of life. We expect perfect health, unimpaired children, freedom from disappointments, and immunity from problems. When the chaos of crisis strikes, when pain, disease, or death come too soon by our own linear standard of time, we call "foul!" But God does not break His own rules. Crises are not evidence of unfairness; rather, they are our personal experience of necessary perturbations within the ultimate order. If we keep calling foul and unfair, it is only because we do not yet understand the game. As you will learn in this chapter, which introduces the eighth secret of science—the power and pervasiveness of life energy—we must learn to see the deeper order of our lives as found in the vibration of the energy of the human spirit.

The Ax of Technology

When our technology goes astray, the victims of this disaster often are advised to "take it one day at a time." I wondered aloud what the alternative was. "Should I have been taking my days in groups of ten or twenty before I got sick?" I would ask sarcastically. "Why isn't life fair? It should be, because God made it."

In fact, life seems unfair when we attempt to "technicalize" and control it by expecting it always to comply with the measurements of machines or the markings on an electrocardiogram. Life seems unfair when our focus on technical "stuff" obliterates our awareness of other realms of reality that do not follow see-and-touch, local rules.

When we cannot correctly set the clock on our own videotape recorder, we may deride ourselves for our inability to speak the right language with our machines. We feel "technically illiterate" rather than acknowledging the limitations that are built into our droning, buzzing creations-turned-creators. The energy state of quantum stuff is silent. Miracle making depends on listening for the tranquility and serenity of energy flowing rather than our machines running and running us.

The ax of technology has cut us off from our awareness of a universal justice and a divine chaos beneath which there exists a miraculous order. We may be shocked, amused, and fascinated by the coincidences and miracles in our life, but they were intended for much more than our diversion and entertainment. Coincidences and miracles are God's attention getters. They offer the lesson that life is fair if we only remember that life operates on an *energy level* that has its own logic and symmetry.

Seeing with Frozen Light

In the "unfair" processes of living and dying, medicine has largely ignored the presence of energy fields and has maintained a strict division between the "hard" sciences of mass and the "soft" sciences of energy forces and the human spirit. My doctors could feel the "particle" me but not my "energy" that held these particles together. By palpating and measuring my body, my doctors could "view" me, but they could not "see me," because they could observe only my physical body's responses.

Science has known for decades that, as physician Richard Gerber writes, "When viewed from the microcosmic level, all matter is frozen light."[1] We are energy fields as much as we are particle people. Yet even when physicians use the principles of the quantum world in their own diagnostic and treatment instruments, such as MRI and CAT scans and laser lights, they continue to think in the see-and-touch world. Instead of asking "Is some *thing* wrong?" they should be asking "How's your energy today?" My doctors and I were so busy trying to find the disorder on a mechanical level that we could not see the energy disruption underlying the chaos of my disease.

The Danger of Seeing Through People

X ray is one example of the way in which energy travels through matter. To assume that the process of X ray does not disrupt the system through which it passes is to ignore the fundamental Fourth Law of Thermodynamics, which states that the flow of energy through a system reorders the system through which it flows. To assume that X ray and other related diagnostic techniques do not alter the system being examined is to ignore the impact of the observer, the tool of observation, and physicist Ilya Prigogine's theory of "dissipative structures," which proves that energy passing through a system drives that system far from equilibrium. Instability results from the act of any observation, and *a new order always emerges*.

Crystals have gained great popularity in the past decade because of the way in which they express mathematic precision through a highly ordered, lattice structure that results in an apparently endless set of edges and valleys. Crystals represent one of the systems of the world that is of the lowest possible entropy, or the least level of falling apart.

Because of the high order of crystals and our sense of that order when we look at them, they have become symbols of healing and spiritual growth. However, when a form of energy is passed through a crystal, disorder results and the crystal may explode into powder. The eighth sacred secret of science is that *energy changes matter and matter affects energy*. Just by the act of examining a patient, that patient's order is altered, and when we shoot X rays through people, new chaos results.

The oldest forms of X ray were "particle" oriented, with X ray tubes placed above the body and a photographic plate held behind. Not unlike the experiments of physicist John Wheeler—described in chapter 6—the patient became the two-slit screen through which the X ray passed. If an "object" interfered with the X ray, doctors saw the disruption on the photographic plate and assumed that some "thing" was "in" there that shouldn't be. None of my X rays indicated that any "thing" was wrong because a type of cancer was growing within me that took the form of waves of energy gone amok rather than solid particles out of place.

As science learned more about energy, it became possible to deal with the patient as a three-dimensional person. Through what is called computerized axial tomography, the CAT scan machine finally presented a clear picture of the source of my pain. During this procedure, a thin beam of X rays is sent into rather than through the patient and the beam rotates 360 degrees. In effect, the CAT scan sees the tissues of the body and the brain from the inside, making diagnosis of growing tumors possible. The CAT scan "feels" and "experiences" a solid tumor from the point of view of the body itself. My tumor was finally detected in this way eight months after my first pain (again the number eight!).

Tragically, I missed my chance for the newest technique that goes beyond even the CAT scan. This was the MRI scan, or magnetic resonance imaging. MRI is a most complicated process, but in grossly oversimplified terms, it works by detecting the slightest energy disruptions anywhere in the body and creating patterns from the chaotic energy of disease. Overgrowth of cells in a tumor always involves such an energy scintillation. Atoms have their own "resonance specificity" or energy pattern, and by studying various resonances, doctors can learn more about cell chemistry and growth. By their own inventions, doctors are moving out of their "fields of specialization" and into the field of dreams of understanding how life energy heals.

I had been scheduled for an MRI test that might have shown my tumor eight weeks after my first pain. Unfortunately, my earlier retinal detachments and the metal clips placed in my eyes from prior surgery made the test a risk to my vision. Because my doctors did not push me to go on with the test and because the machine had been broken on the evening I was scheduled for the test, I decided that the test was not worth the risks. Besides, my doctors were looking for a "lump" and not a "jump." I was only diagnosed when my cancer entered the reality realm of the doctors, producing the sought-for massive lump.

In retrospect, I may have been spared months of suffering and the spreading of my cancer had I risked having the MRI exam. I have learned from all seventeen of my miracle patients, however, that it seems to be a prerequisite to miracle making that one must overcome regrets and realize, as I discussed in the previous chapter, that the past can be altered by our present actions. My advice to anyone reading this who is seriously ill or in crisis is to completely drop any "past regrets" and stop leading what my patients called a "shouldy" life. The way is cleared for miracles by getting into the now.

Watch Out for Zebras!

One of the oldest warnings in medicine is not to interpret symptoms as something major when things usually will "take care of themselves." When I first noticed the pains in my back, I asked one of my first doctors, "You don't think it could be cancer, do you?" He answered, "When I hear hoofbeats, I think of horses, not zebras."

If my doctors had broken free from their local reality realm and looked for several possible explanations for my condition—at least kept an eye out for a zebra on the horizon—I might have been spared two years of agony.

Why Rain Dances Always Work

I met a native Hawaiian dancing on the beach at sunset. He chanted, moaned, and sang as if calling to the whales playing just a few hundred feet away. I watched him for almost an hour, and then he came to sit beside me.

"You're going to ask what I was doing, aren't you?" he said as he pointed to a whale jumping almost completely out of the ocean and slapping the water so loudly that the ground beneath us shook. Before I could answer, he continued. "I was doing an ancient Hawaiian rain dance. We haven't had rain in months. Even the tourists look dried out."

In the typical cause-and-effect orientation of someone still relatively new to the islands, I asked, "Does it work?"

"Oh my, oh my," he said laughing and still watching the whales playing. "You're talking like the middle-aged tourists who come to this middle-aged island to be warmed by that middle-aged star you see setting just over there. You're in a middle-aged hurry. You mean when should you look for results? When should you look for rain? Now, or maybe tonight? Maybe before your visit is over?"

I felt exposed in my profane view of time. I looked down at the white ring around my wrist where my watch had left an imprint from the sun before I finally took it off. I grabbed my wrist to hide the watch mark, and the Hawaiian laughed.

"The Hawaiian rain dance always works," he said pointing out the sudden and brilliant green flash that sometimes happens in Hawaii just at the moment the sun vanishes beneath the line of the sea. "When my ancestors did this dance, it would sometimes work in a few minutes or days or months. Sometimes it was almost a year or two, but the rain dance always brings rain. Sometimes it brings floods."

This underlying order in the apparent local chaos of the universe is the point of all of the sacred laws of science. There is an ultimate order, but that order is a chaotic order of infinite complexity that far exceeds our narrow, cause-and-effect arrangement of the "stuff" and events of our life.

Many scientists take the view of biologist Jacques Monod, who argues that nature has no purpose and that we cannot find and "project our purpose to nature."[2] In the religious camp, Henry

Morris, a chief proponent of creationism (which denies the facts of evolution and advocates a literal interpretation of the Bible), writes that "Order never spontaneously arises out of disorder."[3] These factions each argue from totally divergent points of view, yet they both miss the point that there is a cosmic energy that constantly and chaotically reshuffles the stars of the cosmos and the electrons within us into an order as magnificent as a volcano and as simple as a miracle. In other words, we and our world are spirits in progress, and the energy causing our changing and caused by our changing is infinite.

Aristotle proposed a God that we can come to know by reason rather than faith. He suggested a God based on physics rather than on revelation and wrote about the "unmoved mover" who was the ultimate source of movement and order in the universe.[4] I have found that just as mass and energy are the same quantum stuff, so it is that *both* reason and faith are paths to finding the meaning in life's chaos. I have faith in the order of the universe, and the principles of new science have strengthened that faith. I *know* that spiritual energy exists because science proves it. I *believe* it exists because I felt that energy when I died and returned to heal.

Pain and the Open Gate

In October and November of 1988, my pain was so severe that I groaned through the day and night. A physical therapist attempted to use what researchers call the gate control theory of pain management.[5] I was given a machine with electrodes attached to my hips. Acupuncture stimulation of peripheral nerves in the spinal cord at a level above the entry of the pain was supposed to neurologically "shut the gate" so that pain could not travel up the spinal cord to be "known" by the brain.

The pain machine did not help. I know now that my pain was not in one location. I was experiencing a chaotic energy throughout my entire system, so the local attempt to shut the gate on my pain was similar to trying to block a tidal wave with a few sandbags. The failure of this and other treatments should have forced my doctors and me to explore other realms of reality for explanations, but that did not happen. Instead, we used more and more invasive techniques from within the same mechanical realm.

The sacred secrets of science are secrets only because we fail to apply the uncommon consciousness that would help us see them. Had my doctors and I been more willing to realm hop, we would have found some answers to my problem in the eighth secret of science, which describes the presence of forceful energy fields that surround and heal us.

The Force of Energy

The concept of energy has been central to the study of physics since the mid-1800s. It is a concept used in our everyday language to refer to everything from the ups and downs of our emotional state to the risks of the arms race and nuclear energy to global concerns about our depletion of the earth's energy. (As if the earth's energy is separate from "our" energy!)

Energy, like love, is something we all know and experience, but it is an abstract concept that can't be seen or touched. It is one of the things in our world that we pay for every month, but we never see. Energy and mass are the same stuff: While mass is "touchable and seeable," it really is only a temporary "freeze frame" in the flow of energy. As one of my students exclaimed when she grasped the concept of energy moving in, around, and from everything, "Solids . . . aren't!"

Force is energy's footprint. Force is the push and pull of the cosmos, and it can be measured by seeing how fast an object moves. The faster the object moves, the more force it has. We sometimes confuse these terms: The wise Obi Wan Kanobe would have been more accurate in the movie *Star Wars* had he encouraged the warrior Luke Skywalker by saying, "May the energy be with you."

Energy is the current that charges the chaos of the universe. It is everywhere within, around, and from us. Force is our local experience of energy when we feel pushed and pulled by an energy of living.

A Dream of Fields

Anyone who has worked in an intensive care unit has seen and felt energy fields. "I called them the fields of dreams before the movie of the same name," said Carolyn, one of the nurses who showed her uncommon caring and uncommon consciousness during my treatment. Carolyn would comfort me, clean me, and hold my head and stroke my brow as I vomited in the middle of the night.

"You can see the fields around patients, and you can feel their force," Carolyn told me. They push you and they pull you. They can pull a patient through and push them on. They are real. I don't know why doctors distrust this idea so much. They use fields of energy in the nuclear medicine department all of the time. You're being treated with whole-body radiation, Dr. Pearsall. You're being placed in a powerful field every day, and when you come back up here to the unit, we feel the energy from your procedure. Your body hums."

After Carolyn described these fields to me, I dreamed of them regularly. I dreamed I was back in Maui and I could feel the force of Haleakala pulling me back together again. As I mentioned earlier, hundreds of people had come to Haleakala on August 8, 1988, for a convergence of uncommon consciousness. They were pulled there by what they felt to be the natural energy of the volcano. I know and believe that these healing fields exist.

The Night I Was Spun Like a Top

When my pain was severe, I would lie on my bed in Maui all day and night. I was unable to sleep for more than a few minutes at a time. I would lie with my head raised near the headboard of the bed so I could see Haleakala. For several nights in a row, I noticed a coincidence that was a miracle.

No matter when or in what position I fell asleep, when I awakened, my body would be away from the headboard and centered diagonally on the bed, arms at my sides and legs pressed together. I felt like the needle on a compass orienting toward a magnetic pole. I believe that the magnetic energy of Haleakala rotated me around to heal me.

Einstein said "Belief is more important than knowledge." He meant that faith and conviction are crucial in the attempt to learn about our world. I have never slept in the diagonal position on my bed. I could not even get into that posture when my hips were being eaten away. But the energy of Haleakala arranged me in this healing position while I was anesthetized by my dreams.

I noticed that Haleakala's treatment seemed to take place only on the nights that I dreamed about the energy of that volcano. Was I sensing on some level the cosmic healing taking place? Is there such a thing as healing fields? I know so.

I Was a Middle-Aged Hologram

On the quantum level, energy's dualistic nature of particles and waves makes itself known in every experiment. The Bose-Einstein condensate theory described in chapter 6 suggests that a sudden coherence of energy can cause a "whole" that is much more than the sum of its parts. The type of energy I felt from Haleakala affects every laboratory experiment.

Laser light, a manifestation of all of the aforementioned principles, can be used to produce pictures through a new science technique called holography. Holograms, or the images created by holography, are truly three-dimensional because they contain every part of an image, or the "whole" picture including front, back, and side. Every bit of a laser light carries the entire image of the whole.

If the energy from the light bulb you are reading by (a form of *incoherent* light) were converted to a laser light (*coherent* light working by the principle of a Bose-Einstein condensate), that light would have enough energy to force a hole through a thick steel wall. The power of coherence, of concentrated energy fields, is infinite and it is what I am referring to when I speak of a "life force." Like the hologram, in which every laser particle carries the whole image, *every cell in our bodies carries the energy imprint of our whole "selves."*

When doctors learn to deal with this coherent life force rather than with lumps of life, they will have at their disposal a completely new way of approaching illness and healing. They will be able to help patients learn more about their own "holographic energy template"[6] that controls all of growth, disease, and healing.

The Chernobyl Factor

Following the shock of discovering yet another form of cancer after the diagnosis of the tumor in my hips, I entered the hospital for my bone marrow transplant. Only with this procedure was a total cure possible, because the "sick" energy pattern (referred to as the "clone") of the cancer cells could only be "cured" and reordered through the BMT process. This is the ultimate rebuilding of a holographic energy template, for my own bone marrow was to be taken out, "reenergized" by treatment with chemicals while my entire body was shot with radiation and filled with chemicals to kill any remaining cancer cells, and then put back in to reenergize my body. My bioenergetic pattern maker, my marrow, was going to be altered. I was literally going to be revived in measurable electrochemical terms.

Researchers are learning more about bone marrow transplants every day. The nuclear crisis at the reactor in Chernobyl, USSR, taught physicians much about the removal, treatment, and transplant of bone marrow. Because they had to act quickly to save lives that would never have been saved before, these doctors had to extend their practice of medicine beyond the bounds of their traditional realms. In essence, they had to take their bold technology in both hands and make a leap of faith into a new level of healing.

I interviewed one of the doctors who had gone to the USSR to help in the crisis at Chernobyl. He asked to remain anonymous because he fears rejection from his colleagues for the following statement. "Most of us weren't really sure what to do. These people were killed right down to their marrow. But something just told us to go ahead and do the unthinkable. Take out the marrow. Just do it. Do the right thing. It was like an energy or a message from somewhere telling us to go ahead and that it was the right way to go."

The doctors working in the chaos of Chernobyl were following Patsy's principle. They were going with "the way it is" and responding to what they felt as a powerful energy drawing them toward areas of medicine they had never explored before. The doctor added, "We were like *Star Trek*. We were going where mankind had never gone before, but we were being dragged there reluctantly. Now, as a result, we have a whole new way to deal with and even cure cancer." The same chaotic energy that killed (and will kill) so many at Chernobyl may now result in a procedure of donor and autologous bone marrow transplants that will save thousands of lives. This new order was born of loss and chaos.

Out with the Bad Energy and In with the Good

My first day on the bone marrow transplant unit was actually exciting. My wife and I walked the halls together. Because my first course of chemotherapy had cleared the tumor from my hips and the cells in my hips had been reenergized to generate new bone, I could finally move without the aid of a wheelchair or a walker. I felt a new hope now that one type of my cancer had been defeated and, now that we had made the decision to go ahead with the BMT, my wife and I were like children going through a fire drill. We denied the suffering that we knew lay ahead, and our "enlightened denial" helped us draw on an energy from the realm of the spirit that made it possible for us to continue.

When the doctors removed my marrow and inserted a tube in my chest through which chemotherapy would be given and blood would be taken, the true nature of the procedure became clear. "You think your hips are sore!" said Dr. Joseph Uberti, my doctor who always "made time" to talk and joke with me, "I ground and ground and ground the needles into your bones to get plenty of marrow. We'll purge it and put it back in when your radiation and chemotherapy is finished. My wrists have hurt for days from grinding that needle into you. See what you did to me?"

The doctors could purge my marrow of damaging energy, but they could only hope that a healing energy would return. They could take out the bad, but we would have to trust a higher force to put the good energy back in. There would come that special day when my marrow would be given back and we would all wait for the healing field to do its job.

Treated by a Nuclear Explosion

Once my marrow was removed and stored for treatment, I was given four days of the most intense chemotherapy possible. The marrow had been removed while I was under general anesthetic, but my hips (already sore from the ravaging of cancer) now throbbed with pain from the removal of my marrow. The chemotherapy made me terribly sick. As it had done during my first course of chemotherapy, my hair fell out again. I constantly struggled to remove the hair from my mouth, and would occasionally gag on gobs of hair trapped in my throat during the night. I was stunned to see that this time even my pubic hair was gone. Any fast-growing cell is destroyed by the chemotherapy. Afterward, you can tell when you had your treatment, for like the lines in the trunk of a tree, your fingernails show a "fault line" of disruption and cracking just in front of the new growth. Your skin peels away until a new inner skin emerges.

There was something symbolic about my chemically induced pubescence. I felt that I was being reborn. I was sicker than I had ever been in my life, but I felt more hope than I had ever known throughout this ordeal. I had no energy at all, yet I felt anticipation of a new energy when my marrow would be given back to me new and fresh and clean of disease. I learned firsthand that there is order in chaos, because while my life and body were in total disarray, I felt on the threshold of a new beginning.

Courage by Command

I counted on my physicians to get rid of the bad energy, but I was counting on the prayers and love of my family and friends to replace the sick energy with a healing strength.

"You are so courageous, going through this terrible thing," said one of my doctor friends. "You know the odds of it working aren't so good, and the procedure is one of the most excruciating medical treatments known. You are really showing a lot of courage."

I had seen the courage of the miracle makers whom I had studied. It is a "command courage" because it is bravery born of necessity, not boldness. When we confront our major crises—the necessary chaos in all of our lives—we have no choice but to be courageous. None of my patients has ever shown anything less than tremendous valor even through their most frightening moments. God expects it and sees to it that this energy is offered through the prayers, faith, and loving of family, friends, and healers.

Killing the Cancer Clone

If a bone marrow transplant cures, it cures by providing the patient with cells that are free of the cancer clone mentioned above. The

DNA code provides the growth template for cancer cells. When the unhealthy energy of this cancer clone is purged from the marrow, it is hoped that healthy cells will grow, guided by the healed field of a healthy energy template.

Following the intensive chemotherapy, I was exposed to full-body radiation. I was fitted for a special shield to protect my lungs from the treatment. (The tissue of the lungs is so fragile that my radiation treatments would have burned them away if they had been left without protection.) I was surprised when I saw the clear plasticlike shield in the exact image of my lungs. My lungs seemed so small and frail that I had a sudden flash that something might go wrong with them because of all of this radical treatment. That thought turned out to be a quantum and prophetic leap into my own future.

I then was fitted with a wooden platform that would stop me from crushing my shoulder as I lay motionless on my side during the radiation. I still cannot put on a coat without pain shooting through my shoulders from the long periods I spent lying completely still on my side while I was saturated with radiation. From time to time, I find myself trapped half in and half out of a jacket because I cannot move my shoulders. In effect, I was set up as a sitting duck for a nuclear explosion aimed directly at me.

This mass killing of cancer cells causes terrible side effects that I came to call the "Hiroshima look." There is no pathological human condition that is not caused by this treatment, and the "permission to give treatment" form that I signed listed twenty-five potentially deadly side effects. One statement read, "I understand that I will be given lethal doses of radiation and that this treatment may kill me."

All of us who had been blasted in that dark room (while all the technicians hid in another room) had the Hiroshima look. No hair, skinny, deathly pale from a blood count of almost no red blood cells, completely vulnerable to the slightest germ because nearly every immune cell had been destroyed, always nauseated and hacking with dry heaves, no appetite because the stomach lining shrinks and taste buds are burned away. We experienced almost constant diarrhea because the lining of the intestines is destroyed. Our mouths bled from the radiation burns, but the blood had no taste not only because of the destruction of the taste buds but because blood containing so few cells has no taste. The nurses and our family said that we even smelled burned. We had all been placed directly at ground zero and bombed for four days of nuclear war against cancer with the radiation equivalent of a small nuclear explosion.

I looked around the room where I waited for the radiation to do its job. A long, dark machine was aimed at me. There was one brief click, and then twenty minutes of complete silence in the killing field. I imagined the quiet killing power of this invisible energy field, but I also remembered the principle of complementarity, which would suggest that a complementary silent but powerful *healing* field could also be surrounding me.

I imagined my cancer cells being burned out of me. Then I saw the chairs and tables in the room. This was a place for things that no one wanted anymore. Boxes of stored files lined the room, and large machines skulked unused in the corners. Only the technicians were out of harm's way. I wondered what was happening to the electrons in the tables and chairs. Were they being radiated too? How did they feel? I lay in dead silence while my cancer-ridden body was blasted to a new level of chaos.

When the technicians placed me in position and then left me alone with the machines and furniture, there was an emptiness that could never occur anywhere else in the world. The radiation had effectively taken the energy out of everything in its path, and I could sense this nothingness. The room felt dead, but I felt the spark of life within me. I resolved that I would not join that room. I would escape the battlefront.

Getting Atomic AIDS

The whole-body radiation had done its job. Almost nothing inside me was still alive. I was at death's door. As one doctor told me, "This is the sickest anyone can be and still be alive. Everything is wrong with you and nothing is right. We have almost, but not quite, killed you."

The chemotherapy and radiation were over. Everyone now who even came close to me wore gowns and masks. I had no immunity; a form of atomic AIDS. A chart showing my blood count was placed on my wall. Like a business on the skids, my blood test result line was on the bottom axis. I, my nurses and doctors, my family, and I am certain even my dogs, waited to see if the line would ever go up. If it did not, I would go physically down forever.

The weakness induced by whole-body radiation and intense chemotherapy is not describable. It required several nurses to lift me to be weighed. I could not eat, and the spasms and agony of starving to death had begun. Not until my purged marrow was replaced and would begin to produce healthy blood cells, *if* indeed it ever could, would my stomach be able to deal with food again. There was nothing I wanted; not food, not sex, not people, not anything. Now I knew what my oncologist meant when he spoke of the scorch the earth treatment. I felt as if I had no energy at all, no life energy force other than the life energy of my family and the other healing gardeners around me who were my life energy support system.

All of us waited and prayed for the nonlocal power of our collective human spirit to do its healing work. My medical treatment was over. Almost all that was physically me was dead. All medical efforts were now focused on trying to keep me alive long enough for my bone marrow to come back to life. It was time for the silent healing energy fields to help my soul make its miracle.

The Power of Empathy Energy

On the day the doctors call "rescue" day, the bone marrow transplant team prepared to reinsert my treated marrow. "Aren't you excited?" a nurse asked me. "This is the day you've been waiting for."

"Excitement takes energy," I said. "I have no excitement potential."

I could not think about myself. I had been waiting for results of a biopsy being done on my son Scott on this same day. The doctor had found a suspicious lump in his neck which they thought could be a symptom of the same cancer I had. I could only pray that he would not be found to be sick. Any spark of energy I had was being sent to him.

"Don't cry," said a nurse. "This won't be all that bad." She didn't know that I was crying not from fear of the procedure but in prayer for my son. I bargained that, if only he would be healthy, then I would offer my life in trade.

My wife rushed in. She was exhausted from caring for me, but now she had the added burden of having our son hospitalized for surgery. I looked up, and she said, "He's fine. Just an enlarged gland." I cried so hard that the nurse had to change my gown because of the wetness of my tears. I sobbed so vigorously that every part of me hurt and the blood began to flow backward up my IV tubes. Suddenly, I felt my son sending back a miracle.

I felt a spurt of energy. It was an energy born of mutual empathy, and I know now that "empathy energy" is the strongest healing force of all. I felt my son and my whole family within me, and I could see the hundreds of people praying for me. I felt vibrations through my entire body, and I was in awe of this miracle. I was ready now. The ceremony of the cells could begin.

The Ceremony of the New Cells

The entire BMT unit fell silent. All of the patients knew that a rescue was in progress, and without saying so, the little energy left to the patients was sent as donation to that day's recipient of transplanted marrow. In a scene directly out of a science fiction movie, doctors, nurses, and technicians in huge rubber gloves, long gowns, and masks walked in a long ceremonial line. They were silent, focused wholly on the marrow of life they carried reverently in their hands.

"Are you ready?" said the doctor. No one answered because we all knew that he was asking a much higher power than all of us.

Talking seemed disrespectful of the miracle that was in progress. Hand to healing hand, my purged marrow was passed from its steaming dry-ice container to an "energizing" warming tube that brought the electrons of the bone marrow cells up to the speed of those within my body. The marrow was then placed into a huge syringe. A doctor injected the thick, blackish red marrow directly into the tube in my chest, and I felt that I would explode. "I'm too full," I thought. "I'm going to break open all over everyone."

The newly purged cells ran through my body to find their correct place in the middle of my bones. No doctor knows why or how these cells "know" how to transplant themselves, but they do. The doctors were practicing high-tech faith healing. Just as physicists don't know how "electrons seem to know" where to go and how to get in and out of their orbits, so no one understands the magnificent knowledge of these life-generating cells. All of the patients, doctors, and families must have faith that the marrow will find its way to the deepest part of the bones. There had to be faith that the marrow would recover from its purging on its own, for no medicines were given to help the marrow come back to life in my body. There had to be faith that the patient would recover, for nothing is done for the patient once the marrow is transplanted other than support and the power of prayer. The killing of the cancer is a mechanical process, but the recuperation and healing from the transplant is pure faith.

Everyone could smell a strong garlic odor—the odor of the chemical preservative that had held my stored marrow. My life had been held in suspension somewhere in the basement of the hospital and for some strange reason, I thought at this most unlikely moment, "When I'm cured, I'm going to write my first science fiction novel about bone marrow storage of the great minds and leaders of the superpowers." I even began to construct the entire plot, but was interrupted by another overinflation in my veins and engorgement of my heart as more purged marrow poured in.

As always, my wife was by my side and everyone on the bone marrow transplant unit was silently straining to hear the miracle in progress. If they hadn't known that a transplant was in progress, they could now tell by the terrible smell and the crowding around of doctors and nurses inside and outside of my room. "A tribal healing ceremony," I thought. "Why aren't they chanting?"

The whole ceremony of new cells was over in less than one half hour. As the last injection was completed and the doctors verified that I had survived the ceremony, everyone in the room paused silently. I am certain that everyone was praying, but no one said a word. Every head was lowered, and I saw tears on my doctor's cheeks. Like me, like all of us, he was awed by this closeness to "the way it is" and what it means to make a miracle.

All of us would now wait to see if I would live or die. I knew I would live. The energy of my loving family overwhelmed me as it overwhelmed my disease. Like the radiation that had silently killed my cancer, the silent love energy was now at work. It was invisible, but it was majestic. My son Scott was healthy. Our collective energy was strong. The prayers would work.

Energy Transfusions

In the days that followed my transplant or "rescue," I lived off of energy transfusions. I was given blood transfusions to provide sufficient blood cells to keep me alive until my marrow could provide my own cells, but I also felt that in this blood I took in its donors' spiritual energy as much as I took in their blood cells. More than ever in my life I felt the principle of oneness and nonlocality. I felt the energy being sent to me by my friends and family. I knew the different realms of reality as I felt the see-and-touch world of needles and medicines while experiencing the vibrations of my family's love.

During one of my mess moments when I was sure that my life was over, a parade went by. It was Patsy's parade. She was marching through the halls spreading energy to everyone much as a clown in a parade throws candy to the children. This weak and frail little girl somehow was an energy donor for all of us. Her parade radiated an energy that came to me, by coincidence, at the perfect time.

"Do you want to join my parade?" asked Patsy.

"I can't walk with you now," I said. "But will you let me pretend I'm coming along?"

"Sure," she said. "But tomorrow, you had better march with my parade yourself. You've got to get back in the parade."

As I knocked on death's door, I had the energy to walk away before the door opened completely. I could begin to live because of the energy transfusions from the spiritual donors surrounding me. No matter how much someone mocks you when you speak of oneness, nonlocality, simultaneity, and multiple realities, do not yield to their cynicism, even if their scoffing frightens you and seems to rob you of your hope. I have been a human experiment in total life energy depletion and restoration, and I promise you that healing fields exist and that they surround you now even as you read my words. Can you feel them?

The Spirit of a Salamander

One of the first scientific studies to confirm the existence of growth energy fields was done by Harold S. Burr. A neuroanatomist at Yale

University in the early 1940s, Burr worked to define the shape of energy fields that surround plants and animals.[7] He discovered that the salamander is surrounded by an electrical field shaped much like the animal itself. No one was too surprised by this finding, for scientists knew that all living tissue contains an electrical axis of positive and negative.

As Burr continued his study of the salamander's development, however, he discovered that the plus charge for the salamander's head and negative charge for the tail existed in the unfertilized egg itself. He extended his work to plants and showed that the electrical field of a seedling is not that of the seedling itself; rather, it is the electrical field of the adult plant—a *preexisting energy field growth template* sometimes referred to as bioenergetic growth fields.

Nobel Prize–winning physicist David Bohm writes of the "implicate order," or the idea that there is a holographic universe in which the entire energy of the cosmos is enfolded and coded.[8] That we are directly and immediately affected by an energy template is not speculation; it is scientific fact. It was not always so, however. Much of what was called witchcraft was an attempt—largely rejected by fear, sexism, and the political control of physicians—to acknowledge and use healing energy fields. Because these fields or vibrations could not be seen or measured in the local realm of reality, it was assumed that such fields could not exist. Many healers—almost 1 million women—were burned at the stake because they dared to know and share the fact that we are more than we ever imagined we could be.

Taking a Picture of Spiritual Energy?

At about the same time that Burr was doing his research, Armenian electrician Semyon Kirlian "coincidentally" experienced a sparking between his hand and a glass-covered electrode that he was repairing. Pursuing the meaning of this coincidence, Kirlian and his wife, Valentina, began to attempt to record such "sparking" or electromagnetic fields around living objects. Similar research into energy fields around living things was being conducted almost simultaneously by Czechoslovakian investigators.[9] In fact, the first work on electrophotographic evidence of "energy field discharge" around living things was reported by G. C. Lichtenberg in 1777.

Scientists have long known that there is a universal type of electromagnetic energy given off by all objects called "black-body radiation."[10] Black-body radiation is a basic concept of quantum theory. That a form of this energy could be photographed was another disturbing thought to both science and religion. Scientists were not used to trying to "see" energy, and religious leaders thought it was somehow an indication of weakened faith to attempt to try to "see" evidence of the spirit.

The spirit is real. It is our common life energy. While Kirlian photography has many faults as a research technique, it has offered some interesting insights into the universal nature of energy fields that are a part of all life.

When living objects are photographed by the Kirlian technique of electrography (with high-frequency, high-voltage, low-amperage electrical fields), a corona discharge surrounding the object is seen. This corona discharge is named after the outer corona of the sun observed during an eclipse. Skeptics point out that many factors, such as moisture and temperature, can affect or cause this corona to occur.[11] They assert that there are more than twenty-five physical variables that influence Kirlian images.[12] Although many of the paranormal assertions about the significance of auras detected by Kirlian photography seem to have little merit, several researchers have obtained significant insight into a subject's state of health by reading corona discharge patterns taken from the fingertips.

There are data that certain patterns of electrical corona are related to cancer.[13] There is also some evidence that changes in corona discharge are related to cystic fibrosis.[14] As I have pointed out, no single tool from any one realm of reality can be used to measure all of the dimensions of our life, but one way to understand our existence is through methods that are sensitive to electrical and other energy fields emanating from and around us. Rather than attacking or defending such procedures as Kirlian electrography using only the rules of a realm that may or may not be applicable, we should be busy asking what lessons might be learned about our physical and spiritual realities through these interesting procedures.

The Mystery of the Growing Fields

Why does one plant cell become a part of a kernel of corn and the other a part of the rich green leaf that surrounds the maize kernels? Cell differentiation is a scientific mystery. There is no currently accepted theory that completely explains why one human cell grows into a lung cell and another into a heart cell. The DNA or genetic code for both cells is the same, but something directs them to their final form. Just as electrons are directed to their correct orbit by specific resonances of energy and bone marrow cells are summoned to their correct place by invisible biochemical resonance, so every body cell is responsive to energy templates. Scientists speculate that a factor related to the interaction between cells acts like a growth template, but that factor is not yet fully understood.

In the early 1980s, Rupert Sheldrake, an English plant physiologist, wrote a book called *A New Science of Life*,[15] in which he proposed the existence of "morphogenetic fields." He suggested that these "organizing fields" operate nonlocally, or free of space and time, to make plants and animals what and how they are.

Like Burr's electromagnetic fields that form life from a holographic energy template, Sheldrake's "morphogenetic fields" exert what he called "formative causation," or in the case of human beings, a type of universally existing pattern of growth represented in our collective unconscious.

Sheldrake's morphogenetic fields cannot be seen, but just as in the quantum world, their effect is clear once an observer interprets the field. Like a quantum vacuum, the invisible fields of growth are a spiritual soup from which patterns of realities are created. When we die, the forceful field that collected us into a form moves on, but the cosmic cluster of energy is infinite.

To my doctors, my body seemed useful only as a means of communicating in the see-and-touch domain and interacting with the machines of man's making. For me, my body seemed like a holographic picture of all that I was with everyone, a cluster of energy that some observers chose to see only the see-and-touch aspect of its reality.

The Permanence of Cosmic Clusters

Because religion often personalizes the spirit as "self" rather than viewing it as a cluster of energy, it, too, balks at talk about morphogenetic fields, holographic energy growth templates, and detectable fields of energy revealing themselves as corona patterns. Instead of seeing these spiritual growth templates as God's infinite patterns, religion views them as science's way of explaining God away or diminishing His work.

Talk of energy fields, therefore, is limited to the highest level meetings of nuclear medicine where such talk is necessary because differing realms of reality are being dealt with every day. Only when a new multirealm science is developed combining the principles outlined in this book can there be the merging of science and religion into a healing art.

Energy patterns, or cosmic clusters, are timeless and do not occupy space. Such a form of "existence" is possible because of the principle of nonlocality and oneness. Cosmic clusters are infinite, which makes all of us infinite. These clusters disprove the profane view of our existence as being a fleeting moment with a distinct beginning and complete and final ending.

Playing Host to a Spirit

"Did you ever notice how you can feel a person's presence?" asked Mr. Davies, one of my fellow patients on the bone marrow transplant unit. He was a small, frail man, not over five feet tall. He was just slightly taller than Patsy, who often considered him a potential playmate. He shared with me a love for classical music and often complained about the loud rock music being played by one of the teenage patients on the unit.

"I had a donor for my marrow. I never met the guy, and nobody told me a thing about him, but ever since I had the transplant, I can feel him. There's an energy about it. The doctors don't like to talk with me about it and I suppose it's some type of psychological stage I'm going through in adjusting to my transplant, but I feel the presence of this guy."

"What do you think he was like?" I asked.

"It feels like he was some kind of an artist. Maybe a painter or musician. He played the violin or some string instrument. He was a very strong, a big guy with a lot of power. I can feel his power, but he was an artist, too. He was very gentle. I don't know. It's all so strange."

Weeks later, a medical student assigned to the bone marrow transplant unit was talking with me. He was fascinated with the transplant procedure, and we began talking about donors and hosts, the technical but symbolic name given to the recipient of the donor's marrow. A very serious condition is the host versus graft rejection syndrome, in which the host first rejects the donated marrow and then begins to reject everything in his or her body. Almost as a physical overreaction or startle response to the miracle of new life, the body is overwhelmed. Death can result. Rejection is a complicated process that doctors explain using the chemical concepts of the see-and-touch world.

Although I had received my own treated marrow (called an autologous transplant), I knew that even I had to accept the donation on more than a biochemical level. I wondered why the doctors did not prepare the "host" on a spiritual energy level as well as a physical level, and I asked the medical student what he thought about this idea.

The student dropped his pen. "What do you mean, on an energy level?" he asked incredulously.

"Well, we hosts are taking in the energy of someone else, or in my case a whole new energy system recharged for me by the purging process. My marrow sat there for days being affected by all the energy around it. I wonder how it was treated down there. Were people nice to it? Technically, it is accurate to say that the purging affects the actual bioelectrical field of the marrow, isn't it?"

"Well, yes," answered the student quietly. "But you're talking about more than just that type of energy, aren't you?"

"Yes, I'm talking about energy as a whole because everything is a whole," I replied. "We hosts are receiving all of the energy of the donor or of our own marrow with a new energy, and it might help if we knew more about the nature of that energy."

"No way," said the student. "Usually, it's a family member donor anyway. If not, it should be perfectly confidential. You just need medical facts, as for a sperm donor. The host should not know a thing about the donor. For example, and very confidentially, the donor for Mr. Davies was a big strong macho cop in Detroit. He's nothing at all like Mr. Davies. He plays guitar in a rock band. Why tell Mr. Davies that the guy whose marrow is inside him is so different from him?"

"Even if it is a family member, I still think it would help a great deal to work as much on matching the spirit with the chemistry," I answered, too tired to argue.

Late that same night, I suddenly remembered Mr. Davies's description of his sense of the spirit of his donor. He had described the man as being big and strong, but gentle and artistic. "Was the medical student's description really so different?" I wondered.

By coincidence, at just that moment, Mr. Davies stopped at my door. He was trailing along behind Patsy in her nightly parade. "Hey, Doc," he said. "I found out one thing about my donor. The nurse said she thought his hobby was oil painting. How about that?"

Patsy called to Mr. Davies and scolded him for holding up the parade. As he smiled and moved away, I thought that he had been right on every count. Big, strong, artistic, player of a stringed instrument. Also obvious but not discussed by Mr. Davies and me was the profound tenderness and caring shown by the act of this policeman donating his marrow to save the life of a stranger. Mr. Davies had felt that gentleness, and it saved his life as much as the chemistry of the healthy new marrow. He had experienced a spiritual as well as a physical transplant.

I have often pondered the retroactive effect of the transplanted marrow on the donor. Does the donor experience some bond with the host that is beyond our present means of measurement? If I had to guess based on the principles of new science, I would guess in favor of a strong reciprocal energy relationship between the person who contributes the materials for the making of this type of miracle and the person "hosting" the miracle itself.

The Phantom Spirit

A well-documented scientific finding supports the notion of permanent energy force fields and spiritual energy. Called the "phantom leaf effect," it has never failed to stun my students when I describe it to them.

When the upper third of a leaf is cut off and thrown away, the leaf's bioenergetic growth field remains. If the leaf that remains is electrographically photographed using Kirlian techniques, the amputated part of the leaf appears in the photo and a *whole, intact leaf* is seen.[16] We are all familiar with the phantom limb phenomenon, or the patient who feels pain in an arm or leg that was long ago amputated and destroyed. The presence and lasting impact of growth energy fields is real.[17]

Researcher and skeptic Keith Waner suggested that the phantom effect was due to moisture of the leaf left over on the photographic plates.[18] Using a clear lucite block as a barrier preventing moisture from being electrographically photographed, the phantom image still appeared. The organizing energy fields or Sheldrake's morphogenetic fields are powerful and permanent, working their effects in some realm of reality forever.

Even more remarkable, energy fields have been recorded in three dimensions, even when pieces have been removed and destroyed. In a book describing electrographic photography techniques, it is reported that both sides of the phantom image are detectable and not just a flat, one-dimensional picture.[19] When the remainder of a leaf is electrographically photographed from both sides, both sides of the missing part are clearly seen. The smooth side of the leaf is as apparent as the rougher, ribbed side. Like a three-dimensional hologram, the entire image is detected, providing evidence again of the holistic nature of energy fields.

Rumanian researcher I. Demitrescu used an electrographic scanning technique to examine a leaf in which he had cut a small round hole. The image revealed a perfectly intact, complete leaf *inside* the hole (an exact replica of a leaf within a leaf!).[20]

One of my nurses reported her own personal recording of my energy field. "I can see him healing," said one of my nurses in intensive care as she spoke with my wife. I could hear the nurse, but I could not yet respond. "I can see it and feel it. I can see something like an aura around him, and I see your energy helping to heal him. I've seen it in all of my patients. His is a healing aura. I see it. I know it sounds like I'm nuts, but ask any nurse who has worked in intensive care. They've all seen and felt it."

Crisis Question Number One and a Reenergized Rescue

The same four questions of crisis occurred over and over again during the long and painful weeks of my bone marrow transplant. When I asked the first of the four questions—"Why me?"—I realized that from the point of view of energy fields, I was a "field" as much as a "thing," which made me part of the overall life field. My illness was not "unfair." It was simply part of the constant adjustment and readjustment of the universe. I was a part of the chaos.

My chemotherapy and whole-body radiation had been designed to kill me as a necessary side effect of killing the cancer cells. The host was being "almost" killed so that the parasite had no place to live and grow. This was a necessary part of the energy rearrangement from unhealthy to healthy chaos.

Crisis Question Number Two and the Seven-Year Switch

When I asked "Why now?" I realized that I was ignoring the timelessness of infinite energy fields. We are all always changing, developing, and becoming because chaos is the experience of the constant reordering of the universe. Unless we take a limited, linear view of being born, getting old, dying, and rotting, we see that we are forever changing energy.

Approximately every seven years, we are entirely new. There is not one atom in your body today that was there seven years ago. We all get the "seven-year switch" of our entire atomic structure. I know I am cured not only because of the miracle of the bone marrow transplant but because my newly energized marrow is busy producing new healthy atoms all the time. In five more years, none of the "me" that had cancer will "be."

Crisis Question Number Three and the Need for Energy Transplants

My "Now what?" question was answered from the point of view of our constant need for renewed energy. What I had to do when I was dying was to merge with and receive the transplanted energy of those around me.

I remember wishing that I had received a donor's bone marrow instead of my own. I thought that, even though the risk of rejection is higher in such cases, I would get a newer, less-selfish energy by getting someone else's marrow. "I've always been so self-sufficient, and even now when I'm dying, I'm getting a transplant from me," I said. Then I realized that I was not seeing how I could receive my transplanted energy on a much broader scale.

I could allow myself to merge with the energy of those who love me. Loving is a form of reciprocal energy field transplant. I noticed that, when all of the visitors were gone for the night and only the patients and staff were present, the energy seemed to be running down on the BMT unit. The patients' energy was low to begin with, and the staff was being drained constantly by the patients' need for their energy.

Our loving visitors brought with them the energy we so badly needed. Even when the visitors themselves did not come, those patients who were open to the principles of nonlocality could receive their energy transfusions by long distance. The hundreds of family pictures and furniture brought from home were energy in the form of "mass" or particle, but they held within them the energy waves of their loving origins.

Crisis Question Number Four and Feeling Fields

When my energy seemed completely gone, and the taking of my marrow, the chemotherapy, and the radiation had drained me to near empty, I knew more than ever that we all share one common energy field. The answer to my "So what?" question was that we are indeed as much orbit as electron, as much energy as particle.

More than at any other time in my life, I could feel the energy fields of those around me as I began to lose my grip on life. I learned that my energy depended on the energy of everyone else. I learned that we share one eternal energy that, as in the leaf-within-a-leaf experiment I described earlier, is represented within each of us and shared among all of us. Today, I am still hypersensitive to energy fields and can sense energy disruption. My wife complains that I have become "field finicky."

"You're like someone who smoked for years and quit and now is so sensitive to smoke that they drive everyone crazy," my wife said. "You're getting to be field finicky, and some of us just aren't as sensitive as you are right now."

After I gave a speech in San Francisco recently, when people crowded around, I noticed that I could exchange a quick glance with certain members of the crowd and know, "You've made many miracles, haven't you?" I have never been wrong when I ask that question. We recognize each other by the energy around us.

Connection and the Silversword

Maui's official flower is a tiny pink rose called a lokelani. It makes beautiful floral leis, and when we have visitors, we greet them at the airport with leis of lokelanis called bozo leis.

The unofficial flower of Maui, however, is the silversword. The name silversword in Hawaiian is *ahinahina*, which means "gray gray." This particular plant can be found only on the slopes of Haleakala above the 6,000-foot level. Hundreds of them surround the Haleakala crater edge itself. The silversword lives for almost thirty years and ends its physical life by sprouting gorgeous stalks of hundreds of purplish red flowers. As the plant ends one phase of its reality and its ethereal energy moves on, it celebrates this transition through its floral explosion. Then it becomes a nine-foot-tall gray skeleton symbol that continues to be beautiful, natural, and energizing. These plants are never *pau*, the Hawaiian word for "ended."

These wonderful plants are protected now. It is a federal offense to damage them. It is seen as *kapu*, or "forbidden" to touch a silversword. Laws had to be passed because these plants are so powerful that tourists are drawn to them and want to take them home.

During my last trip to my home in Maui, I met an old Hawaiian man who was serving as a part-time guide at Haleakala. He was sitting several feet away from a cluster of silversword plants. He was a *kahuna*, or a "wise and healing elder" of the islands, and he was sitting there being reenergized by the plants around him. The Hawaiians have known the energy we share with nature from the beginning, and all of their gods represent the spirit of God in everything.

"I've seen them begin to shrivel up just by a bunch of people with cameras running at them," said the *kahuna* ranger, talking softly so as not to offend or embarrass the plant. "I've seen them bend and cry in fear just like a *keiki* [child]. I've seen them drained of their magic energy by the *haoles* [tourists]."

He paused to look up at the sun, then looked back at the plant as if attempting to relay some new energy. "But I've seen them flourish when certain people are near. The quiet, peaceful, gentle person who stays their distance seems to give the plant energy. It's the loud, insensitive, aggressive people who are the energy leeches. They make Maui feel very bad, and his plants weep."

As the *kahuna* spoke, I could feel his own healing energy. I sat with him and felt the power of the silversword several feet from us. We were both quiet for a few moments, and my miracle and the silversword caused me to cry.

"You're *kamaaina* aren't you?" he asked. *Kamaaina* is pronounced "comma-I-na" and is Hawaiian for "a new child of the land." It is a word used in Hawaii to refer to native-born Hawaiians or residents who have "transplanted" to Hawaii and become renewed as compatible parts of the Hawaiian culture and the spiritual mythology, legends, energy, and natural beauty of the islands.

Startled by the similarity between my bone marrow transplant experience and my *kamaaina* status, I responded without thinking, "Yes, I'm *kamaaina*." The lessons of my illness, my near death from cancer and its treatment, and my transplant had awakened me to the deep spiritual connections that unite us with each other and with the cosmos, transcending chaos, crisis, and death.

My wife was seldom away from my side through every day of my hospitalization for my bone marrow transplant. Even though I would sleep for hours, she would sit by my bed. I could feel her energy even in my sleep, and I would awaken if she left the room. To pass the endless hours, she would put together jigsaw puzzles with pictures of flowers, trees, streams, and the sun in the sky. Somehow, in some way, she seemed to be putting me back together again through her unifying and loving energy.

The eighth sacred secret of science that I have documented in this chapter—the existence of forceful fields—requires our constant attempt to "connect" with the energy around us to find meaning in chaos. When we connect, we behave in a way that respects our ultimate relationship with the universe. By learning to pay attention to the influence of energy fields in our lives and to the miracles and coincidences that signal their constant presence, we discover the ultimate fairness of life. Life is fair, but the fairness is an awesome, nonlocal fairness that transcends our simple, mechanistic sense of justice.

In the next chapter, we'll explore the principle of "divine dynamics" as one of the forces of fairness in the universe. As it turns out, we are not falling more and more apart; rather our lives become reorganized through crises and miracles. When we can call on this faith in the ultimate order and meaning of chaos, we are well on our way to making our miracles.

NOTES

1. Richard Gerber, *Vibrational Medicine: New Choices for Healing Ourselves* (Santa Fe, NM: Bear, 1988).

2. Jacques Monod, *Chance and Necessity* (New York: Alfred A. Knopf, 1971).

3. Henry M. Morris, *The Troubled Waters of Evolution* (San Diego: Creation-Life Publishers, 1975).

4. Aristotle, *Basic Works*, ed. Richard McKeon (New York: Random House, 1941).

5. R. Melzack and P. Wall, "Pain Mechanisms: A New Theory," *Science* 150 (1965): 971–979.

6. The concept of a holographic energy template being the road map for the growth of the fetus and the healing of the body is described in medical detail by physician Richard Gerber, *Vibrational Medicine*, 51.

7. H. S. Burr, *The Fields of Life* (New York: Ballantine, 1972).

8. For a description of the concept of "implicate order," see J. Briggs and F. Peat, "David Bohm's Looking-Glass Map," in *Looking Glass Universe: The Emerging Science of Wholeness* (New York: Simon & Schuster, 1984).

9. S. Prat and J. Schlemmer, "Electrophotography," *Journal of the Biological Photography Association* 7, no. 4 (1939): 145–148.

10. Details of this type of radiation are presented by physicist Harold Morowitz, *Cosmic Joy and Local Pain* (New York: Charles Scribner's Sons, 1987), 126–128.

11. The many factors related to electrical corona and electrography are reported in W. Tiller, "Present Scientific Understanding of the Kirlian Discharge Process," *Psychoenergetic Systems* 3, nos. 1–4 (1979).

12. J. O. Pehek, H. J. Kyler, and D. L. Faust, "Image Modulation in

Corona Discharge Photography," *Science* 15 (1976): 263–270. See also W. W. Eidson, D. L. Faust, H. J. Kyler, J. O. Pehek, and G. K. Poock, "Kirlian Photography," *Proceedings of the Institute of Electrical and Electronic Engineers Conference* (Boston, 1978).

13. S. Mallikarjun, "Kirlian Photography in Cancer Diagnosis," *Osteopathic Physician* 45, no. 5 (1978): 24–27.

14. These data are in a report that was published in the periodical *Medical News*, Mar. 6, 1978, 24. Further speculation about the relationship of corona discharge patterns and illness and wellness is found in R. Gerber, *Vibrational Medicine*, 53–54.

15. Rupert Sheldrake, *A New Science of Life* (Los Angeles: Tarcher, 1981).

16. This phenomenon has been repeated hundreds of times and is described in "Ghost Effect," *IKRA Communications* (June 1978). See also T. Moss, *The Probability of the Impossible* (Los Angeles: Tarcher, 1974); K. Johnson, *The Living Aura* (New York: Hawthorn, 1975); and T. Moss and K. Johnson, "Radiation Field Photography," *Psychic Magazine* (July 1972): 50.

17. Further elaboration of the "phantom energy effect" is found in S. Krippner and D. Rubin, *The Kirlian Aura* (New York: Anchor, 1974); and S. Krippner, ed., *Energies of Consciousness* (New York: Gordon & Breach, 1975).

18. Reported in Thomas Moss, "Puzzles and Promises," *Osteopathic Physician* (Feb. 1976), 1:30–37.

19. Thomas Moss, *The Body Electric* (Los Angeles: Tarcher, 1979).

20. I. Demitrescu, "Life Energy Patterns Visible Via New Techniques," *Brain/Mind Bulletin* 7, no. 14 (1982).

10

THE PROOF OF IMMORTALITY

Getting It Together by Falling Apart

> When something doesn't go my way, I let go of my idea
> of how it should be, trusting that my mind doesn't know
> the larger picture.
>
> —ELIZABETH RIVERS

> I'm growing old! I'm falling apart! And it's *very interesting!*
>
> —WILLIAM SAROYAN

Haunting My Own House

Breathing faster did not bring me any more oxygen. I could not catch my breath. Just moving my body caused me to gasp and struggle as if I were drowning in a sea of air.

I had survived the bone marrow transplant and returned home, but I felt like a visiting spirit in my own house. Everything looked familiar and brand new at the same time. I felt the reverse of the common *déjà vu* sensation of visiting someplace new but feeling as if one has been there before. I was visiting the place where I had lived for more than a decade, yet I felt as if I were here for the first time.

I wondered if this was how a ghost feels as it moves through its former surroundings. My dogs looked at me and whimpered as if I were something going bump in the night, and my family seemed awkward and unsure of how to relate to me. Even as I sat inches away from him, my son would ask "Does Dad want to eat anything? How's he feeling?" He was trying not to bother me, but it felt like further evidence that I wasn't really there. It was like I was haunting my own house, sometimes startling a family member or a dog accustomed to my immobility by actually walking through a doorway.

The life force I described in the previous chapter had nearly left my body, and it still did not feel like it was securely locked back within me. There seemed to be two "me's": a physical and a spiritual me trying to get back together again.

Friends were not allowed to visit because whole-body radiation had rendered my immunity almost nonexistent. Even plants were not allowed to visit me because they might contain spores that would cause an infection. I was supposed to stay alive by avoiding contact with life. I was not supposed to have dogs in the house for fear that I would catch a doggy disease. My wife had the dogs shaved to the skin and sterilized with surgical soap, but it was still a risk that my doctors found very unwise. I needed as much spiritual energy around me as I could get, however, and the dogs seemed a minor risk in my efforts to reunite my body with my soul.

My stamina was so low that I could not breathe well enough to talk for long on the phone, and I noticed that it seemed to be becoming more difficult to breathe at all. I could not pay attention to reading or television or even conversations with my family. I could not seem to feel whole, connected, and vitally alive.

Sexual Spirits

I had been concerned that the radiation and toxic chemicals of my therapy might be transferred to my wife's system through any sexual intimacy. My attempts to get medical answers to this question were unsuccessful, but it was in part through sexual intimacy that I eventually began to feel human again. The touching, holding, and intensity of orgasmic experience seemed to be one of the first ways that I "came back together."

Months after I had begun to reunify my body and spirit, I was talking with Pete, the native Hawaiian gardener who takes care of my Maui home landscaping. He had read one of my earlier books, titled *Super Marital Sex: Loving for Life*,[1] and was teasing me about the sexual prowess of the demi-god Maui. "You know," said Pete, "that Maui was a sexy dude. He caught the sun by its genitals with a rope he made out of the pubic hair of his sister. Then, he was finally killed by a goddess who squeezed him to death with her legs when he tried to crawl into her vagina when she was sleeping." Pete laughed, but he had the legend exactly right according to the books about Hawaiian mythology.

"The spirit is real sexy," said Pete as he hacked away with a machete at some palm leaves that had served their purpose of keeping their plant alive and now had lost their life energy. "You know you aren't here no more when you don't feel sexy," he said as he laughed. "You want Pete's sex book? It's better than yours, Doc."

"It's very simple, *Blalah* [brother]," said Pete as he paused to wipe the sweat from his forehead with his forearm. "Buy when your blalahs is selling, sell when they is buyin' and make plenty *aloha* [love] the rest of the time." Pete laughed loudly and went back to work, but the simplicity of his philosophy had been a key to my own recovery.

Locked Out of the Energy Field

Before I became whole again, the invitations to lecture had stopped, and publishers were not calling to ask about my next book. Even when I felt my energy returning, I felt locked out of the overall energy field of the general world.

As I have pointed out, there is an infinite energy field, but this energy has to be engaged with the body in order to present itself in the local world. Neither the energy growth template nor the physical body itself remains together for long when death occurs. In the phantom leaf experiment described in chapter 9 in which a missing part of the leaf leaves an energy imprint even after it is gone, the phantom effect does not last for long. Similarly, the physical body is the local advertisement of the spiritual presence, and when that body is finished, the spiritual energy reorganizes to other levels.

I had almost died several times during my scorch the earth

treatment. My doctors and I had counted on my ethereal template and holographic energy field described in chapter 9 to hold on until my physical body could reform and join it to make a spiritual and physical whole. My spirit was waiting for my body. The connection was not yet complete, and I may be one of the first scientists who has been a ghost.

I drifted in and out of alertness. My family said that it was "like Dad just disappears on you." I bumped into chairs and walls as if I were trying to go through them. I did feel that I could pass through solid objects because I did not feel solid myself. I was almost all wave and only loosely organized particles.

When I first saw a picture of myself taken at this time, I was shocked. I had been a tall, athletic, skinny man with boundless energy. Now the chemotherapy had ravaged by body. I *looked* like a ghost! I was gaunt, emaciated, pale, and had no hair. There was no life in my eyes, and I was bent over like a very old man.

As I continued to sort through the pictures of me as a ghost, they showed a body almost beyond use, seemingly being dragged around by a spirit that refused to let it go. I cried at what had happened to the physical shell that held my spirit. I didn't know it then, but I would soon know again profoundly and exactly what it feels like to leave my physical body. I would soon learn that it is faith and unquestioning belief that accomplishes the ultimate reordering and getting it back together again.

The Gecko Syndrome

As I was writing the words above, a coincidence has just happened. My wife just cried out, "Oh, now look what I've done. I shut the door, and this poor little gecko got its tail cut off."

A gecko is a small lizard found all over Hawaii. They are a symbol of good luck, and their little bodies are capable of an echoing, scolding chirp that can be heard for several hundred feet. Their image is found on many of the thousands of T-shirts that threaten to weight the island back down into the sea. Their *tsk, tsk, tsk* scolding seems always to be heard when we need to be slowing down to live in the *aloha,* or "loving spirit," of Maui. We have learned to listen to and respect the gecko as a type of "monitor alarm" of our life pace on Maui.

"I feel terrible," said my wife, stooping to look closer.

The gecko was fine. He would regrow his tail. Like the salamanders mentioned in chapter 9, he was surrounded by his electrical energy growth template that would regenerate his tail to join his body. "But look," exclaimed my wife. "His tail is still moving without him!"

The tail still held a part of the gecko's life energy. In a few minutes, however, the energy had no complete vehicle in which to travel. The tail stopped moving, but the gecko had moved on to sing again that night. The gecko syndrome, the organizing and regenerating of life energy in and out of the physical vessel of the body, is an example of the ninth sacred secret of science to be reviewed in this chapter—the Second Law of Thermodynamics and related findings about energy. It was this sacred science principle that was making itself felt when I went through my experiences as a ghost and learned that falling apart and back together again is a part of the necessary chaos of our existence.

Orderly Apes and Obstreperous Atoms

Once, when I was lecturing about the relevance of the Second Law of Thermodynamics to healing, one of my first-year medical students seemed completely puzzled. She was not used to realms other than that of biology being used in medical science.

"I don't have the slightest idea what the Second Law of Thermodynamics is or what in the hell it has to do with healing and living," she said. "I don't even have any idea what the *first* law is! Is there a first law, too?"

The First Law of Thermodynamics states that energy is always conserved; it cannot be created or destroyed. Energy and matter are the same "stuff" revealed in dynamic lumps and jumps, but all the stuff that is or ever will be in the cosmos was created in one Big Bang.

The Second Law of Thermodynamics holds that the quantum lumps and jumps or "stuff" have existed since the Big Bang in the form of an isolated and closed energy system that will eventually burn itself out. The process of moving more and more toward maximum molecular disorder is called entropy, which is the scientific term for a constant falling apart.

These two laws are as valid today as they were at the time they were formulated in the mid-1800s at the very same time when, by coincidence, several scientists were working out the principles of evolution and the concept of ever-increasing order in the universe. Biology was suggesting that we seemed to be falling more and more together, while physics was predicting that we were falling more and more apart!

Are we, as the Second Law suggests, gradually falling apart? Or, as Charles Darwin suggests, are we constantly evolving toward a higher order?[2] Are we ever-evolving apes or a collection of tumultuous atoms in a constant state of disarray? When I was a ghost, was I getting a glimpse of my ultimate disappearance or was I experiencing a chaotic order of the assembly and disassembly between the physical and the spiritual realms?

Ecologists all over the world are now changing their view that the normal condition of nature is equilibrium.[3] Plant ecologist Stewart Pickett states, "The balance of nature makes nice poetry but not such great science."[4] Studies of the forests, climate, and atmosphere of our earth reveal that turmoil is the natural state of nature. The quiet forest is actually a sea of turmoil, including the death and rebirth of hundreds of plants and animals in a chaotic dance of beautiful turbulence. George Jacobson, a paleoecologist, writes that while there may be a tendency toward a stable equilibrium (Darwin's view) "it's never allowed to get there, so we might as well not expect it to exist."[5] Through my experience as a ghost, I have learned that the "falling apart" described by the ninth secret of science (the Second Law of Thermodynamics) is the natural phase of our living, and that any negative or positive order we see in our daily lives is always a *tendency* and never a *final* state. Even Darwin's evolving apes experienced their changes through a random and often chaotic shuffling of genetic mutations. To become more orderly apes, atomic disarray is necessary.

Making a Beautiful Mess

The apparent contradiction between natural order and cosmic entropy can be resolved by remembering the existence of multiple realities. In contained, laboratory-controlled experiments, everything does in fact move toward disorder. Laboratory experiments, however, take place only on one level of reality and in isothermal-energy–burning (isothermal meaning isolated and thermal) systems. The Second Law of Thermodynamics correctly predicts and explains the nature of such closed and self-contained systems.

Living biological systems, however, are not closed. They are reactive to a vast environment of stimuli and are constantly growing and changing through a constant state of turmoil. While entropy always increases on the local see-and-touch, contained level, in the realm of our human experience, entropy is merely a shuffling to a new "chaotic order." "Order" does not necessarily follow our linear, local definition of being "perfect and complete and organized." Chaotic order implies a beautiful imperfection, a challenging and patterned incompleteness, and a glorious disorganization.

This chapter focuses on these times of transition to and from chaotic order: what I call the "tendency times" of our remarkably beautiful way of falling meaningfully apart. We will explore the neguentropy, or movement toward chaotic order, of open life systems and show how this variation on the theme of the Second Law of Thermodynamics applies to the making of miracles.

A Tendency Toward the Miraculous

The Nobel Prize–winning physicist Ilya Prigogine proposed the term *dissipative structures* to describe the fact that when systems are driven far from thermodynamic equilibrium, they become unstable and then spontaneously organize themselves in a much different order of a much larger scale.[6] If as observers we see only the "tendency times" of instability or transitional local order, we think that our world either is in beautiful balance or is a complete mess. In fact, our world and our life is neither magic nor mess; it is pure "tendency." The sense that everything is just right or all wrong that we experience every day is an illusion conjured up by a process of chaotic order far beyond the simple local examples of a neatly kept house or files arranged in perfect alphabetical order or the apparent chaos of a messy house or a serious illness.

The Laws of Thermodynamic Medicine

The concept of chaotic order has far-reaching implications in treating illness. If we realize that the Second Law of Thermodynamics proves that disorder is natural and necessary and accept that the entropy of disease is, like all things, a part of the whole of our existence, we will stop trying to fight disease and begin trying to understand how disease works as a form of ultimate healing of the collective human spirit. All individual suffering is really the local experience of cosmic change and reordering. Disorder is as necessary for a healthier form of order as great volcanoes were to the formation of the paradise of the Polynesian Islands. Our pain is not diminished by our knowledge that our experiences are a part of the evolution of our larger human spirit, but our fear can at least be reduced by the sense of some meaning in the chaos of our suffering and the understanding that there is ultimately much more than here-and-now discomfort and distress.

I ask my medical students to remember that there is also a Third Law of Thermodynamics that, while not spoken of often because it applies to the entropy of pure substances in the rare atmosphere of absolute zero, may hold one key to the healing arts of the future. The Third Law reminds us that in *our* daily lives, nothing is perfect or pure. Uncertainty is a fact of the process of trying to know and to cure. We must never be completely certain about a diagnosis. We should be open to the process of learning not only what but why something is "wrong" (i.e., causing chaos in the body). When we are dealing with the human body and mind, we are not dealing with a pure system, but one destined for a chaos that has a purity (as Prigogine suggests) far behind our present grasp.

Finally, the Fourth Law of Thermodynamics suggests that it is the flow of energy through a system that brings order to that system. We must not forget that healing energy—not mechanical readjustments alone—constitutes true holistic medicine, and we must try to be energy donors rather than energy leeches.

When I teach this little lesson called "The Laws of Thermodynamic Medicine" to my first-year medical students, they always wonder about my sanity. After a challenging question-and-answer period, however, some students always come to my office to ask questions about God, time, and the meaning of the universe.

"If God is so smart, why did he create this mess?" my students often ask me.

I answer, "It took God to create this wonderful chaos. You're just a contributor to that chaos. Just try to see the chaos and learn from it instead of fearing it. Don't see chaos as God's mistake. Instead, see it as God's gift of creating higher and higher order. See chaos as a manifestation of what I now have come to call Patsy's principle, or 'the way it is.' "

Again we are faced with another choice concerning a local versus a nonlocal view of life. Either we see the universe as a re-verberating, infinite system revealed to us through a series of dis-ordered movements toward a more majestic and still mysterious chaotic form of ultimate order, or we see the universe as created with a Big Bang only to expand until it burns out with a small sizzle to a black hole of nothingness. I have chosen the former alternative, and if I needed any more convincing, my journey from life to death and back again strongly reinforced that choice.

Almost Dying Again

Although I was finally home after eight weeks in the hospital, I still had to make periodic visits to the transfusion center. Wearing a surgical mask to prevent exposure to a germ that could kill me, I was taken by my wife to this frightening place of a dozen large lounge chairs lining the walls. Several patients would be sitting there receiving blood transfusions to boost their blood count sufficiently to at least keep them alive. Frail, pale, and bald from our treatments, we would each wait our turn to have our blood taken to determine whether or not a lifesaving transfusion was necessary.

"You're doing fine," the nurse assured me.

"But I feel terrible," I answered. "I'm just not me. I can't eat, I can't think, and I can't even sleep. Nothing is like it used to be. I feel like a ghost. I can't move my left shoulder, my left thigh hurts, my hips still ache, and I feel so terribly weak."

"It's typical of a bone marrow transplant patient," she attempted to reassure me. "You've been through a lot. Just give it time. Your energy will come back."

The energy did not come back. In early November 1989, I began to die. I struggled to breathe, and my wife took me for tests. A large tube was forced through my nose and into my lungs to look for the cause of my breathing problems. A pulmonary function test was done, and the technician yelled at me to "blow all the air out so

I can see how much air you can hold!" Try as I might, I could not blow. A small razor was used to slice my wrist to take blood from my artery to measure my blood gases and thus assess the efficiency of my lungs. My lungs, once strong and elastic from years of playing the saxophone, could not seem to expand. I felt the panic of not being able to get oxygen.

At this same time, my wife's doctor had discovered another suspicious lump in her breast. We went to a surgeon who inserted a needle into the lump to determine if the lump was malignant. I could only huddle helplessly in the corner of the examination room, offering the energy of my presence and wondering about the pointless disorder of it all. Then I remembered the quote by physicist Harold Morowitz: "Given the wonder of the universe, it seems wrong to focus on its alleged pointlessness. Existence is point enough; everything else is a bonus."[7] At least I was existing, and I prayed that just that fact would help my wife now.

I could not warm myself. I shuddered uncontrollably, and I could not move without feeling dizzy from the lack of oxygen. I couldn't think or speak clearly because of the lack of oxygen, and now I was fearful for my wife's life. Before the doctor completed the test, he excused himself for an emergency phone call. "I'll be right back and we'll see if this thing is cancerous or not," he said.

I thought about the famous thought experiment devised by one of the founders of quantum theory, Erwin Schrödinger. He hypothesized about a cat placed in a cage of solid walls with radioactive material, which has exactly a fifty-fifty chance of causing death— depending on the direction of the particles that would be emitted. If the particles go up, poison goes into the cat's food and the cat dies. If the particles go down, the cat's food will remain unchanged.[8] According to quantum theory, the cat is both alive and dead, just as "stuff" is both wave and particle, until an observation of it is made. The particles make their moves, but until we look, nothing is certain about the fate of the cat. Once we look, the cat is either dead or alive. Now, as we waited, my wife did and did not have cancer at exactly the same time. It is our observation that creates the reality.

Once again, my wife and I found ourselves waiting together for news. The doctor finally returned and made his observation of the lump. In about the twelve seconds it took him to say the words "It's just a cyst," our life was changed again. "See, no problem," he said. I thought, "If you only knew the problems we still have."

A Rush to a Rescue

"He's not responding to anything we're doing," said the doctor. "I'm afraid we're losing him. We'll have to do a lung biopsy. It's risky now to do surgery, because he just finished his transplant, but we have no choice. He's slipping away from us."

Two days after I had waited with my wife to find out her fate, my condition had become life threatening. I was hospitalized and my wife and the nurses were crying at my side. An oxygen mask was placed over my nose and mouth, but still I could not get sufficient oxygen. The Life-Pak, or electrical paddles that contained the invisible energy that might be needed to reestablish a better order to my heartbeat, were placed on the cart beside me. Doctors and nurses ran, pushing me down the halls to surgery.

Out of the corner of my eye and just over my clouded oxygen mask, I saw my wife, one of my sons, and a police officer friend of my son's who had driven him to the hospital. They were all trying to hide their tears.

I said, "I love you. Don't worry, We'll make it." What is remarkable is that I seemed to know that I would make it, even though the murmurs of the doctors and nurses were to the contrary. "He doesn't have much longer," I heard one doctor say. "Is he still alive?" said another. I could see me being pushed down that long tunnel as if I were hovering over the entire scene. Later I would be able to recall every sound and sight of my near death.

Getting the Spirit Back In

When I awakened from anesthesia, I could not move or open my eyes. As I reported in chapter 1, I was dying but I was aware of everything around me and felt as if I were levitating within the intensive care cubicle. When my family's tears joined mine, they provided a flood of energy that seemed to reunite my body and spirit. Like the salt water of the ocean around Maui, the salty tears seemed to carry me back to the see-and-touch world, and I knew I would be here in Maui writing this book and telling you about this miracle.

"Wait until they read this," I remember thinking. "This will make some story. I wonder if anyone will believe it?"

Three tubes had been inserted in my chest, and the biopsy of my lung had revealed that a common virus called the cyto-megalovirus was rapidly turning my lungs to rigid cellophane incapable of processing oxygen. Bone marrow transplant patients do not typically survive this type of infection. It is a viral attack called "the forties" because about forty days after transplant, patients in their forties may experience an oxygen level of less than 40 percent in their blood. That level causes a state of borderline death. I heard the doctors in the operating room say, "I don't think he'll make it through the night. He probably will never come out of this anesthesia."

I chose to come back from death. The peacefulness, safety, and seductive feeling of freedom I described in chapter 2 as being common to most near-death experiences was strong, but something told me that I had to come back. I felt myself being "returned" and reassembled. I felt the energy fields around me doing their healing work, and like the regenerative gecko syndrome, I was becoming whole again. I could actually feel the vibrations of healing like the tingling you feel when your foot becomes numb because of poor circulation. I felt the power of my family's energy transfusions and the power of my friends' prayers. I was being vibrated back to physical life. At long last, I felt my spirit merging with my body.

The "Bad Bunch" Phenomenon

Suffering, it seems, always involves several bad things happening at the same time. There seems to be a universal law of "bad bunches" that plagues persons in crises. Like me, my seventeen miracle patients all asked the same question: "Why does everything bad seem to happen at once?"

I have never known a miracle maker who didn't suffer, and I have never known a miracle maker who didn't have to deal with several problems at one time. Although my wife didn't tell me during the time when I was so near death, just prior to leaving for the hospital for her vigil over my surgery and placement in intensive care perhaps never to come home again, she had listened to this message on our answering machine: "I'm sorry to have to tell you this over the phone, Mrs. Pearsall, but I just have been unable to reach you. There is evidence that you might have cancer of the colon. You need a colonoscopy immediately." As my wife sat with me, slept through the night with her head on my chest, and gave me her repeated energy transfusions, she carried the private burden that she, too, might have cancer.

There is an explanation for what might be viewed as a fifth crisis question of "Why all of this at the same time?" The answer rests with another finding from new science called the principle of resonance.

Getting Out of Tune

Everything seems to go bad at once because the vibrations are bad. The concept of "bad vibrations" has received bad press through its association with the marginal cults of pseudoscience and pseudoreligion, but the resonance principle is a proven scientific finding that explains healthy and unhealthy vibrations. When the vibrations are "entopic," the whole system quivers in disarray. Like a symphony orchestra with just one violin terribly out of tune, the entire orchestra begins to lose its harmony as the musicians grapple with their instruments in search of the right tone. Similarly, when all things seem to be going badly, it is because we have, at least temporarily, lost our "healing harmony."

The Harmony of Healing

The resonance principle maintains that the electrons within an atom occupy specific energy shells or orbits. Each orbit is characterized by a specific frequency of energy or its own resonance, and electrons dance to the music of this resonance, moving orbit to orbit only if they are tuned to the exact energy of that given orbit. When an opera singer hits just the right high note to shatter a wineglass, she has matched perfectly the resonant frequency of that glass.

Because we, too, are made up of electrons, we vibrate and resonate in accordance with the energy around us. The electrons of which we are constituted are exactly the same as the electrons of a chair or the string of a violin. When there is a change in frequency or an incompatibility of frequencies, electrons begin to jump from orbit to orbit.

When everything seems to be bad at once, our life is out of tune and the music of the cosmos has gone flat or sharp. When everything is harmonious, everything seems to go right and fall into place. Just like the Bose-Einstein condensate demonstrates the suddenness of the occurrence of a coherent whole, life is played in a major, well-tuned chord. A system for understanding how this attunement works on a spiritual level is found right here in the Hawaiian Islands where I am, by coincidence, writing this book.

The Journey of the *Kahuna* Healers

One of the most significant coincidences in my life, and one that would help save my life by reminding me of the principles of healing and the making of miracles, was my discovery of the mythology of *Huna*.9 *Huna* is Hawaiian for "secret." The *kahunas* who practice *huna* were among the very first miracle makers. *Huna* is an ancient Hawaiian religious, spiritual, psychological, healing system that was practiced until the missionaries took over the islands in 1820—an event that was foretold by the *kahunas*.

The rich verbal history of the native Hawaiians reveals that long ago, there were twelve tribes living in the lush and fertile greenness of what is now the Sahara Desert. The *kahunas* practiced their psychoreligious system in this paradise now turned desert. They believed in pantheism or the presence of God in everything and everyone, as written about by Spinoza and accepted by Einstein.

Through their skill at uncommon consciousness, the *kahunas* foresaw that their Sahara paradise would dry up. They moved their tribes to the valley of the Nile and built the Great Pyramids. The *kahunas* sensed a coming time of darkness and despair and a challenge to their belief in our oneness with God. They needed a place to begin again, to heal, and to renew.

Using the remote vision I referred to in Chapter 6, the *kahunas* saw beautiful uninhabited islands in the exact middle of the Pacific. For their place of healing, they chose this newly created place that had just suffered the chaos of its volcanic birth. They navigated by the stars, including the cosmic cluster of Maui's hook or Scorpius.

Huna is based on the Hawaiian concept of *mana*, which means "spiritual strength" or, in our new science terms, a type of Bose-Einstein condensate. *Mana* predates with almost complete accuracy the concepts of cosmic and quantum science.

The *mana* force operates on three levels, similar to the differing realms of reality. In the *Huna* system, these three realms were called *aumakua, uhane,* and *unihipili,* or the "high, middle, and lower" domains of existence. The *kahunas* believed that a universal substance—a type of quantum "stuff" called *kino-aka*—existed that was both energy and thing at the same time and constituted the etheric substance of the cosmos. This closely resembles the dynamic nature of matter and energy described by the wave/particle duality theory of quantum science.

The three *Huna* realms use *mana* differently. The local, here-and-now self called *unihipili* uses simple and basic *mana* and follows the rules of our everyday, see-and-touch world. The higher realm of reality, *uhane,* uses *mana mana,* the more powerful energy of healing and of daily, meaningful miracles. This is the force that helps the *kino-aka* (or, in the words of modern science, the energy growth template) form for the development of our physical body. Finally, the highest domain of the collective self, *aumakua,* employs *mana loa,* the energy of the entire cosmos. This is the power that generates the magnificent miracles of our life.

I discovered the books describing *Huna* during the same summer of 1988 in which I had first felt the pains in my back. The date, in fact, was near that special August 8, 1988, date on which many religious groups scheduled meetings at special "cosmic power places" throughout the world where the *mana* or spiritual energy was the strongest. The most powerful of all of these places was *Haleakala* on the island of Maui, the dormant volcano just above my Maui home whose lava forms the foundation of my house.

Hundreds of years before the work of Sigmund Freud and his theory of the three structures of personality, the id, ego, and superego, the *kahunas* spoke of the three levels of the self as *unihipili, uhane,* and *aumakua.* Hundreds of years before the work of Semyon and Valentina Kirlian in 1950 in Russia on the electrography of coronas of energy around human and plant bodies and the work of Albert Einstein and Max Planck in cosmic and quantum science, the *kahunas* knew about the quantum stuff of *kinoaka* that is the aura of life. Every major theory of new science was understood by the *kahuna* in Hawaii. As Mark Twain so accurately pointed out, "The ancients have stolen all of our best ideas."

I read all of this material about *Huna* with great interest even as my pain worsened, but I did not then connect it with the sacred secrets of science that I am writing about now. When I returned to Maui to heal, however, my book on *Huna* was sitting on top of my computer. The woman who helps to take care of our house in Maui found it lying on the floor. She said, "I think Haleakala knocked it off your shelf. It wanted you to read it. We had another quake, and that book fell out."

The *kahunas* had found a way to find meaning in their chaotic world of volcanoes, tsunamis, hurricanes, earthquakes, and winds so strong that the natives had to tie themselves to the palm trees to save themselves from being blown into the ocean. They understood that local disorder is only a "transition time" toward a cosmic chaotic order. This was an understanding that I sorely needed.

Haleakala's direction that I study *Huna* again and rediscover its proof of the spiritual and scientific truths of the cosmos was one of the most meaningful coincidences of my life.

A Loving Language of Healing

Even the Hawaiian language reflects an awareness of energy resonances. It is based on resonance and vibrations of sound that the *kahunas* feel translate to the spirit. The *kahunas*, or "healers," chanted for health as well as to sing with the mountains, trees, flowers, and the sea. They believed that the vibrations of the palate, located just below the base of the brain, caused the lower brain to vibrate. The lower brain, sometimes called the reptilian brain because of its seniority in our brain's evolution, is the seat of our most basic emotions.[10] The *kahunas* thought that "good chants" could cause good vibrations by reverberating through the palate into the lower brain, causing beneficial changes throughout the entire brain and eventually in the mind and the spirit. The famous psychologist B. F. Skinner asks, "Is the mind what the brain does?"[11] If we can make our brain vibrate, perhaps we can help the brain resonate to wellness.

There are only twelve letters in the phonetic Hawaiian alphabet. Hawaiian is a way of speaking and singing at the same time. Unlike the arrhythmic English language, which spits, sputters, and cuts off several sounds, the Hawaiian language flows and hums. *Mahalo* is the melodious Hawaiian for the abrupt-sounding English phrase "Thanks a lot." Perhaps if more of us chanted and sang rather than threatened and swore, we would be in better tune with "the way it is" in nature.

Negative Entropy and the First Crisis Question

When I was dying, my agonized questioning of fate often caused me to groan and swear—far from the *Huna* ideal. "Why me, Lord, why me?" ran through my mind countless times. I couldn't breathe, and my "Why me?" question took the form of an angry, desperate demand.

I remembered Patsy's principle, and her statement about "it's just the way it is." I realize now that in our local, immediate suffering and pain, "the way it is" appears to be a process of entropy or falling apart. In the larger sense, however, we fall apart as individuals as a means of falling together as a collective spirit.

The Second Law of Thermodynamics operates in daily life. Everything is moving through disorder. Our illnesses and crises are the personal experiments that prove this law. We are not being singled out for agony; we are moving through and toward a chaotic order of meaning and permanence of our soul.

"Why Now?" and the Second Law

When we listen to the gorgeous complexity of a symphonic fugue and hear the initial theme being reintroduced in several variations and harmonies, we do not ask, "Why now?" when a new variation is heard. We trust that the music has its own logic and pattern that will unfold if we allow ourselves to be taken by "the way it is." We do not try to tell the composer what to do. At times, as we listen to a complex symphony, it seems that everything is a musical mess as the conductor waves frantically to guide the orchestra through disorder. The violins are playing one theme, the wind instruments another. Finally, an ultimate order emerges with a sense of coherence as the energy of the music and the spirit of the composer combine in a resounding finale. Even after the pattern of one composition is completed, however, another piece always remains to be played, and we will be taken on yet another adventure through chaos and "the way it is." The last symphony will never be written or performed, because music, like life, is always being created and composed.

Nor is there one right time for the passages of disorder. We could not enjoy an evening at the opera if a singer came out, sang two lines of one song of sorrow, and then left the stage as the curtain fell. We would feel incomplete. We need *all* of the chaos, pathos, humor, and tragedy to make a full and meaningful performance.

"Now What?" and Patsy's Patience

The "Now what?" question often is a panic question. It is born of trying to put all of the pieces together quickly without having a clear idea of what the whole puzzle is supposed to look like. As my wife often did, one of the patients on the bone marrow transplant unit was almost constantly working on a jigsaw puzzle. She worked at it for hours, and it remained unfinished on the table for days. Nurses and doctors could not resist stepping over to fit a piece in. The puzzle had 15,000 small pieces, but they created no picture. The puzzle simply depicted a beautiful and unique blue of various shades.

"How can you stand to work on a puzzle like that?" Dr. Death Vader asked her one evening. "There's no picture."

"I just enjoy the process," she answered. "Even if I do finish it, I just take it apart again anyway. Just like my life. Put it together and it ends up apart. The pieces just pile up back in the box in their own order when I'm done putting them in my order."

This woman did not survive her transplant. I remember her family boxing up an incomplete puzzle left on the table by her bed. "She loved these things," said her daughter. "It seemed to give her comfort to try to put things together. It never bothered her that she didn't finish a puzzle. It was like her life. She really enjoyed the doing."

The "So What?" Question and Energy Going Everywhere

If we accept the ninth sacred secret of science—entropy as a divine dynamic leading to a chaotic order beyond our narrow local view—we come to understand that the crisis question "So what?" is answered by "because there can be no order without the process of disorder." Suffering is as necessary to our spiritual development as celebration.

"I led an organized, structured, careful life, and now look at the mess I'm in," I lamented. "I'm dying. All of that effort at making a life has all gone for nothing." This is our emotional experience of entropy. All of us feel it at some time in our lives. I felt that *my* efforts at imposing *my* order on *my* life should have guaranteed a constant state of health. I was not seeing that it is not "my way" that is the template for the order of the universe; it is Patsy's principle of "The Way." As diligently as I may work to maintain order in the see-and-touch realm of reality, cosmic and quantum realms of reality have their own "ways."

"Things were very good then," my wife answered. "They'll be good again. Life is fair, but it just doesn't *seem* fair when you're in the messy part of the fairness. Things will get organized again, if we work on seeing the new organization. We just haven't been able to see the pattern yet. You couldn't have seen Maui when it was an erupting volcano. We'll see a totally new way of living for us that comes out of this." I learned through my suffering that I have married a *kahuna*, and my wife, Celest, was given the perfect cosmic name for her healing and loving energy.

The "new way" is the underlying mysterious order in the evolving chaos of living. Our local suffering is but one small vibration in the overall harmony of our cosmic joy.

Faith in False Gods

Faith is the technique that helps the ninth sacred secret of science contribute to our miracle making.

"I have plenty of faith," said one of my students. "I just don't know what to have faith in. That's why I go to the Grateful Dead concerts. I guess I have faith in them. They are chaotic in their concerts. They tune up right in front of everybody and they just mess with the music. But they're always there and they sing about things that mean something to me. I feel more together after I've been through their chaos."

This student experienced what some researchers call the "Lennon Syndrome." This syndrome suggests that we first learn to have faith in our parents. Then we have faith in mystical figures. Eventually, we develop a faith in whatever our peers seem to be having faith in at the moment. Rudolph Valentino was worshiped by repressed young women seeking an outlet for sexual feelings that could not be expressed in the sexist world. James Dean became a source of worship and a role model for young people seeking relief from the restrictive 1950s. John Lennon was worshiped as a god of defiance and noncompliance with the status quo.

The Lennon Syndrome is not limited to performers. When I lectured recently in Rome, I saw "Pope on a rope" soap models of Pope John. I even saw a pizzeria advertising "Pope pizza." This type of worship reveals our yearning for faith even though we, like my student, often are unsure of what to have faith in. We have very low "tendency toleration," and are eager for an immediate and simple order.

No matter what your personal religious beliefs, there is one unifying principle that can provide a sacred faith: We actually help create ultimate order by our faith in that order, because we create our ultimate reality through our chosen perceptions (observer participantcy) about our world.

I have learned to "have faith in faith." The sacred principles of science that prove the survivability of the human spirit across time and space are proof that our faith is better placed in a God of chaotic order than the solid but false idols who provide a quick, local "fix" when everything seems to be falling apart.

A Miracle Drug at the Miracle Moment

"Can you hear me, Dr. Pearsall?" asked the doctor. I nodded my head. I was fresh out of my most recent near-death experience, and the doctor was outlining my next course of treatment.

"We have a coincidence here," he said. "Just days ago, the Food and Drug Administration approved a new medicine. It's called gangcyloverin. At exactly the time you got that cytomegalovirus, this drug was approved for use. When you were dying, we went ahead and tried it on a mercy basis. It seems to be working well. You'll go down in history with your miracle cure. What a coincidence. What a miracle. But there is one big problem."

Once again the flash of about twelve seconds of hope and fear went through me. "We know that the drug can work in some cases, but it tends to kill bone marrow. You just started getting your marrow back, and we don't know if this drug is safe for you. Also, we don't know how much or for how long to give it. We'll have to guess and take a risk, if that is what you want to do."

I remembered the gambler syndrome so characteristic of my seventeen MMs and so crucial to my decision to go ahead with my bone marrow transplant. I recalled our inclination as described by psychologist Carl Jung of allowing our fate to be determined by the metaphorical turn of a card of coincidence. The coincidence of this miracle was strong, and I decided to go with it. I would take the risk with the new drug.

"We have no idea how much more of the drug to give you. There are no guidelines at all," the doctor cautioned. "You've had quite a bit of it already."

At that moment, I thought of Maui. I remembered August 8, 1988, the date when my pain started. I remembered that I had become engaged to my wife on the eighth day of the eighth month and that my son had won his kindergarten contest by guessing the number eight. I remembered that spiritual leaders congregated at Haleakala because of the powerful coincidence of the series of eights in 8/8/88. I recalled that, during my own courtship when my wife and I wanted to say "I love you" over the phone when our parents were nearby, we used a secret code of saying the number eight for the eight letters in "I love you."

"We have decided to try twenty-one more days of treatment just to be safe," said the doctor as he stood up to shake my hand to congratulate me on my survival.

I refused to let go of his hand. "No," I said. "I want eight more days of treatment. Then, I'm going straight to one of the eight major islands of Hawaii. I'm going to Maui."

"Why eight more days?" asked the doctor. "You've almost died. You can't just take off and go halfway around the world!"

"Why twenty-one?" I countered. "And yes I can. I'm here today, but I'm gone to Maui. In my spirit, and in eight days, I'm gone to Maui." Weeks later, I sent this doctor a picture of myself and my family taken on Kamaole Beach in front of my house. The card read, *Aloha! Maui no ka oi* ("Love, Maui is the best")." I had sensed I could have faith in the strange and inexplicable order evolving in my life, manifested by the coincidental but meaningful clue of the number eight. My faith in that larger order allowed my lifesaving miracle to unfold completely, restoring me to health after the chaos of cancer. I signed the card with the number eight to thank the healing doctors and nurses, or in Hawaiian, those *kahuna lapaau* who had helped me to make a miracle.

NOTES

1. Paul Pearsall, *Super Marital Sex: Loving for Life* (New York: Doubleday, 1989).
2. By coincidence, other scientists were speculating about exactly the same evolutionary principles as Darwin at the same time. See Charles Darwin, *On the Origin of Species by Means of Natural Selection, or the Preservation of Favoured Races in the Struggle for Life* (1959).
3. William K. Stevens, "New Eye on Nature: The Real Constant Is Eternal Turmoil," *New York Times*, July 31, 1990, pp. C1–C2.
4. *Ibid.*, C1.
5. *Ibid.*, C2.
6. G. Nicolis and I. Prigogine, *Self-Organization in Non-Equilibrium Systems* (New York: Wiley, 1977).
7. Harold Morowitz, *Cosmic Joy and Local Pain* (New York: Charles Scribner's Sons, 1987), 203.
8. For a more complete and less simplistic review of Schrödinger's thinking about a nonlocal mind and the interaction between consciousness and scientific study, see Erwin Schrödinger, *What Is Life? and Mind and Matter* (London: Cambridge University Press, 1969). See also Schrödinger's *My View of the World* (Woodbridge, CT: Ox Bow Press, 1983).
9. For a complete description of this ancient Hawaiian form of healing, psychotherapy, and spiritual belief, see Enid Hoffman, *Huna: A Beginner's Guide* (West Chester, PA: Whitford Press, 1981).
10. The three levels of the human brain—reptilian or basic emotional area; mammalian or the stress management area of the brain; and the neomammalian area or cortex of the brain—are described in Paul MacLean, "On the Evolution of Three Mentalities," in *New Dimen-*

sions in Psychiatry: A World View, vol. 2, ed. S. Arieti and G. Chrzanowki (New York: Wiley, 1977). The relationship between these three mentalities and health and healing is described in P. Pearsall, *Super Immunity: Master Your Emotions and Improve Your Health* (New York: McGraw-Hill, 1987).

11. B. F. Skinner, "Can Psychology Be a Science of Mind?" *American Psychologist* 45, no. 11 (1990): 1206.

11

CELEBRATING CHAOS

The Miracle Within the Mess

It turns out that an eerie type of chaos can lurk just behind a facade of order—and yet, deep inside the chaos lurks an even eerier type of order.

—DOUGLAS HOFSTADTER

Let us again look at the laws of thermodynamics. It is true that at first sight they read like the notice at the gate of Dante's Hell.

—JAMES E. LOVELOCK

Chaos as Cosmic Coursework

There is no darkness as complete as the Hawaiian night. Two thousand miles from any mainland and free from the ambient light that usually brightens an evening sky, there is only jet black background for innumerable sparkling specks of white glittering over the islands. On this night, I sat with one of my neighbors on our back *lanai*, or "porch." The stars seemed to be flowing out of the crater at the top of Haleakala. "Look at the billions of stars," he said. "Exploded all over the place all over the universe. What a fantastic cluster of cosmic stuff."

My neighbor is a retired airline pilot. He had seen hundreds of black skies with billions of stars. He had learned, just as the *kahunas* had, how to navigate his way in part from reading locations of the stars and planets. Now, as he took a less pragmatic and mechanical view, he was awestruck by the wonderful randomness of it all. "One Big Bang, and cosmic stuff got strewn all over everywhere," he said leaning farther back in his chair. "Just a cosmic chaos, and we're just a tiny, insignificant part of it all."

My neighbor was right in seeing the cosmic chaos, but wrong in assuming that we are an insignificant part or external observer of this chaos. The new science of chaos theory teaches that even the smallest part of the cosmic whole becomes amplified into a majestic order. All of the oscillations of the cosmos contribute to the chaos, but the chaos is not without predictability or beyond comprehension. Discovering its order and meaning represents the ultimate challenge to our uncommon consciousness as we matriculate through the cosmic chaos curriculum. Only if we see students as being insignificant to learning are we insignificant observers of a pointless, disorderly universe.

The key principle of the tenth secret of science—chaos theory—is that *the smallest variation or vibration in the universe results in a complex chain of changes throughout the entire system*. Immensely complex but extraordinarily beautiful patterns always result from just one minor but cosmic and quantum modification. Chaos is a form of order that requires faith as much as appreciation, for we must trust that our existences, our sufferings, and our celebrations are something more than random vacillations in a pointless and ultimately ruined world. We can celebrate the fact that we are able to experience the struggle to understand the tendencies of a higher order. We are capable of trying to comprehend "why we are." That miraculous capability alone is proof enough that there is meaning in chaos.

Scientist Steven Weinberg's *The First Three Minutes* is a lengthy account of the events during the first 180 seconds after the Big Bang.[1] It is a brilliant description of the initial oscillations that would result in the chaotic order we live in today. He states, "The more the universe seems comprehensible, the more it also seems pointless." I suggest that Dr. Weinberg has mistaken chaos for "pointlessness," and that the immenseness of this chaos is point enough.

We need, however, to have patience with our level of cosmic understanding. Our 4.5 billion-year-old planet is located in a 15 billion-year-old universe. Our physical bodies have been here at least as long as the Hawaiian Islands, or 2 million years, but we have been thinking about who and why we "are" for only about 10,000 of those years. We are just beginning students at soul school, and like all neophytes, we are overwhelmed at our place in the chaos.

Most of us will be enrolled in the physical curriculum of soul school for about 70 years. The physical soul school itself is scheduled for total destruction in a burning cinder in about 8 billion years. As individuals, we only have our three score and ten to grapple with chaos, but the new science of chaos teaches that everything, including us, is a key and necessary contributor to that ultimate chaos. Who knows how developed our uncommon consciousness might become over the next 8 billion years of soul school? We still have approximately 114,208,529 individual lifetimes left in which to develop our collective consciousness!

Einstein once was touring an observatory and wondering at the remarkably complex telescope. "We can see stars so far away that they are as old as the universe. We are just insignificant specks on this one little planet going around one little middle-aged star," said the chief astronomer.

"I used to think we were just trivial specks, too," said Einstein, "Until I remembered that the speck is important enough to be allowed to be doing the looking and thinking."[2]

This story illustrates the significance of our participation in the universe. It is easy to feel our place in the cosmic chaos when we celebrate, but it requires strong faith, uncommon consciousness, and a loftier sanity to keep making miracles when we are suffering through the crisis tendencies of the chaotic chain.

Chaos as Character Builder

From August 8, 1988, when I first felt my back pain, to December 8, 1989, when I left the hospital after my near-fatal bout with pneumonia, I had survived more than sixteen months of excruciating pain, two cancers, three major surgeries, multiple painful tests and tubes shoved down my throat, a bone marrow transplant, a week on total life support, the possibility of cancer in my son and wife, school problems for my other son, two chemotherapy courses, extensive whole-body radiation, what was thought to be certain death in intensive care, a lecture tour to Rome, a lecture tour of the west coast, and the writing of a book. I had experienced thirty-two weeks of total chaos, but my life had more meaning than ever before. I learned that life means experience in learning to celebrate chaos.

The ninth secret of science—the principle of entropy—had slammed into my soul, but I sensed that the entropy or movement toward disorder that I felt daily in my illness and treatments was, in fact, movement *through* chaos: a dynamic momentum, not a passive victimization.

My suffering had liberated me from the shackles of constantly striving for a see-and-touch order of feeling good and being healthy. I no longer had to try desperately to interpret what seemed to be the randomness of the cosmos in my attempt to navigate a narrow, local, and ultimately terminal path through my life. I no longer had to "fight my disease" or "struggle to get better."

I was free to learn and to "be" rather than just to "do" the mechanical dance of trying to get my life straightened out, fixed up, or put in order. I understood that *everything that happens tends equally toward being both a mess and a miracle.* That left me free to be me instead of being a patient fighting a disease.

Divine Dissipation

I came to see the extraordinary order of chaos as the ultimate health, embracing the pain of falling apart as well as the wonder of being able to know and feel the divine dissipation surging through me. I could see that the extent of my suffering was possible only because it was this same chaotic energy that allowed for the celebration of my joy.

I experienced how one almost invisible cell can multiply in milliseconds to eat away my bones, and that the whole process began with one chaotic swirl in the energy growth template within that tiny cell. I took comfort from the power of malignancy, because it also taught me that healing has this same mysterious power and happens the same way: through tiny but significant changes in my uncommon consciousness.

I could feel literally in the marrow of my bones the surging patterns that constitute the chaos of the human spirit. My local suffering caused my cosmic celebration because I now had a new meaning for order. With that meaning came freedom from the constant pressure of trying to understand and force a surrogate order out of the infinite tendency toward a chaotic whole.

Joseph Ford, a leading theorist in chaology, points out that evolution is a form of chaos with feedback. Science writer James Gleick writes, "The universe is randomness and dissipation, yes. But randomness with direction can produce surprising complexity. And as Lorenz [a chaos theorist who studied chaotic patterns in world climate] discovered so long ago, dissipation [falling apart or local disorder] is an agent of order."[3] "Randomness," in the view of the science of chaos, represents the flickers of an evolving new order.

Joseph Ford answers Einstein's famous statement that "God does not play dice with the universe" by pointing out that "God plays dice with the universe. But they're loaded dice. And the main objective of physics now is to find out by what rules were they loaded and how can we use them for our own ends."[4]

Something Always Has to Go Wrong

Perhaps the one principle of daily living that no one can escape is that, sooner or later, something always goes "wrong." Anything that does not fit our cause-and-effect view of order has "gone wrong." To assume that going wrong is evidence that the universe is moving toward an ultimate "wrongness" or disastrous end is to ignore the chaology finding that the small anomalies, quirks, and coincidences of life are the necessary sparks and evidence of movement to new order.

Going wrong is the ultimate means for setting things right—so long as we learn a new view of "right." *Right* is not healthiness, happiness, and organized living. Right includes disorder as much as it includes what appears to us as order.

Are earthquakes, tornadoes, tsunamis, and predatory killings in the wild "wrong"? Or are these chaotic events microcosmic oscillations of the developing spirit of life? They are, in fact, the horribly magnificent jolts within the lithosphere, swirls within the atmosphere, swells of the hydrosphere, and crises within the biosphere. As a mere seventy-year student in an 8-billion-year educational program, it is difficult to see such a big picture when we ourselves feel like such a small part of that picture.

Daisies, Deserts, Albedo, and Libido

There is a glorious patterning to our existence in everything from the shapes of snowflakes, the ebb and flow of the depth of rivers, and the patterns of climate, politics, and the falling in and out of love happening all over the world. Everything from a traffic jam to the unique curvature of a toenail is a manifestation of the order of chaos.

Scientists James E. Lovelock and Lynn Margulis proposed what they call the "daisy world" model for explaining how chaos represents order.[5] The word *albedo* refers to "the ratio of the light reflected by a planet to the amount of light that it receives." Lovelock and Margulis theorize about the rhythms of life through their description of white daisies, which reflect light to make our planet cooler while black daisies absorb the light of the sun to make the planet warmer. A third color, the red of the unplanted desert, results from the mixture of various plants that thrive because the *albedo* (or ratio of light absorbed and reflected by the earth) is maintained by the dance of the white and black daisies.

Paradoxically, white daisies thrive in warm weather, even though they themselves help make the planet cooler. Black daisies need a cooler temperature, even though they are major contributors to keeping the planet warm. The apparent chaos of cooling plants requiring warmth and warming plants requiring coolness is a part of the overall order of albedo. The drama of give and take, gain and loss, heat up to cool down and cool down to heat up, goes on infinitely. The order of this chaos cannot be seen if we look only at the life of the single daisy.

Psychologist Sigmund Freud defined libido as a form of psychic and sexual energy that we invest in our living and loving. We may fall passionately in love and become "hot" for a person who is exactly the opposite of the type of person we need for a mature and growing relationship. Then, when just the right person for us comes around, we may become "cool" and reflect them away. It's our hope that we learn and develop *through* the chaos and pain of loving and losing. Through openness, vulnerability, and trust, we learn to love maturely. This usually means striking a chaotic order in our personal lives between our hot and cold love patterns so that a dynamic love results.

When we are going through a "love crisis" or falling in or out of love, things seem unfair. Our lives seem chaotic and we feel alone and deserted. We think that this turmoil will end in frustration and perpetual isolation. The chaos view of love is that this albedo—these patterns of taking in and pushing away—is the order of love and living, just as illness and wellness are both key parts of our "chaotic health." Love aches as much as it invigorates because loving and losing are two sides of chaos.

How Pete and I Saved Millions of Lives

In the last thirty-two weeks, I have lectured to more than 15,000 people, completed two books (including this one), and along with a "plant healer," I have just finished saving millions of lives. So much order has come with my chaos that I feel totally disorganized and am loving every minute of my present mess. I have learned to "seize the moment" and grab on to all of the chaos I can.

When we arrived at our Maui home, our entire landscaping was burned to yellow brown. The rainbow of reds, oranges, pinks, creams, and purples that had dotted the deep blue-green of our hedges, lawn, and trees was gone. The landscape looked as drawn and sick as I had looked in that ghostly picture taken of me during my treatments.

Millions of blades of grass, plants, and flowers were dying. They needed an immediate miracle, and we went to work. Fertilizer was spread everywhere and I watered every inch of our property by hand. Hour after hour, I sat on the lawn surrounded by the beautiful natural features created by the chaos of Haleakala's eruptions. I saw the west Maui mountains and the islands of Linai, Kahoolawe, and Molokai, each created by the chaos of passing over the tectonic "hot spot" deep in the ocean. Now, after all my suffering and healing, I was attempting to be a healer of the natural flora around me.

The lithosphere, the soil, regained its nurturing strength while the biosphere, the plants and trees, responded to their respective growth energy fields. The hydrosphere, the water and the warm afternoon showers falling from the clouds caught and held by Haleakala just long enough for a healing bio-bath, urged the plants to grow again. The warm evening air, the atmosphere, protected the healing plants during the cool night, maintaining a perfect albedo. But none of these factors seemed to be sufficient to make the miracle. The plants still were not flourishing.

"What we need is a plant *kahuna*," said my wife. "We need a specialist in intensive caring for flowers."

Just when I was most discouraged about the meager response of our plants, I heard a cracking sound. I looked over toward my neighbor's house, and I saw a large man pruning wild and thorny bushes with his bare hands. These were the bougainvillaea plants that sparkle with color throughout Hawaii. Their sprays of bright multicolored bracts grow quickly in Maui and throughout my neighborhood. The thorns on these bushes are sharp, but this man did not have a scratch as he gently broke off branch after branch.

I walked over to speak with him. As he talked with me, he kept working. His name was Pete. He was born on Maui to a native Hawaiian mother and Caucasian father. He had golden hair and a beard to match, both of which seemed sometimes to merge with the glare of the bright afternoon tropical sun. He agreed to come to my house and diagnose the turmoil of our plants.

"*Auwe!*" said Pete, in pidgin, a language of Hawaiian mixed with English. *Auwe* is pronounced "ow-way" and means "too bad." "No worry. We make it *mobettah* ["more better"], *Blalah* ["brother and friend"]. When Pete is *pau* ["finished"] it will all be *mobettah*. We get the *keikis* ["babies"] in order." We had found the counterpart of the plant lady who had been gently tending plants in the doctor's waiting room when my crisis had begun. We had found our plant *kahuna*.

"*Mahalo nui loa*," I said, meaning "Thank you very much."

"*No mek mention*," Pete replied ("You're welcome, don't mention it"). He made the traditional hang loose sign with both of his hands held up, thumbs and little fingers extended, with the other fingers in a loosely clenched fist.

"Tight and loose at the same time," I thought. I was working on this book and had just finished writing about the duality of waves and particles and the patterning of chaos. This hang loose sign of closed fist and open hand at the same time seemed a perfect symbol.

Pete provided a fifth realm of reality—a nosphere—for healing our plants. He created a spiritual atmosphere for them: He stroked them, talked to them in Hawaiian, walked singing and without flinching through the cold water of the lawn sprinklers to adjust a sprinkler head. He worked for hours in the heat; then stood fully clothed under our garden hose and showered himself.

I thanked him and asked how much I owed him. "Eight dollars an hour," he said. "The number eight again," I thought. Laughing, I paid and thanked him. "What you laugh about, *Blalah*?" he asked with a broad smile. I didn't explain this coincidence, but he seemed to understand it. He never counted the money. He simply shook the water off his body much the way a dog who has just played in a pond quivers the water away. "*Aloha*," said the plant *kahuna*, and I knew that we had made our miracle. Like the millions of plant lives around me, I was healing.

Poison Plants and Tidal Waves

As Pete continues to take care of our landscaping, he has taught me many lessons. One lesson particularly is a clear example of the science of chaos. Along the rear of our property are dozens of huge oleander plants standing almost fifteen feet in the air. With their white, cream, pink, rose, red, and coral flowers sprouting from their slender, pointed, dull green leaves, they blow in the trade winds like green versions of the blue waves hitting the shore on the beach in front of our home. We had them planted years ago because we had seen them on a drive to Hana town, said to be the demi-god Maui's favorite place.

Hana town is often referred to as "Heavenly Hana," for it is a beautiful, secluded spot reached only by a treacherous, chaotic, and winding drive to get around the protection afforded Hana by the slopes of Haleakala. Some local people feel that the name "Heavenly Hana" comes less from mythology than it does from the relieved cries of the frightened rent-a-car tourists who finally make it there and shout "Thank Heaven! We made it to Hana."

When I told Pete about how we had found our oleander amid the beautiful seclusion of Hana, he explained that the oleander is deadly poison. If one were to eat food cooked on a plate that had held oleander, he said, he would very likely die. Birds and insects will not go near it. He said that the plant was like Hana and like all of life: beautiful and ugly and always changing.

Pete told us that the oleander plants that were so beautifully poisonous reminded him of a crisis that had occurred in beautiful Hana almost thirty-five years ago. An earthquake in the Alaskan Aleutian Islands sent huge 100-foot-tall tsunamis, clocked traveling at more than 500 miles per hour, looming toward Hana. The waves came roaring one after another to overwhelm the town. "Hundreds of Hawaiians were taken away in the watery arms of death," said Pete. "Everything is good and bad, but the tourists, they only see one Hana now. They don't know of all of Hana. Like your oleanders, there is always poison and beauty." Pete knew that the chaos of our life means that there is always a snake in Eden and that all good has its necessary evil opposite.

Tsunamis come just after the ocean withdraws hundreds of feet from shore. Everything becomes still, and the bottom of the ocean is exposed by the suction of the impending tidal wave. Sometimes, people rush unaware to collect the huge seashells exposed by the hundreds of yards of receding ocean. Then, suddenly, with a thunderous rumbling, a towering wall of water more than fourteen stories high rises up and crashes over the shoreline, reaching up into the hills to wash the people away.

Any single phase of the chaos of a tsunami does not give the full picture of the order within these tidal waves. An earthquake half a planet away occurs, a large but imperceptible swell surges through the ocean at hundreds of miles an hour, the water sucks back from the shoreline from the force of the impending doom, and the waves strike to kill and destroy. It is horrible and it is magnificent. It is all necessary and it is all, like my crises and yours, a form of order that can be as totally overwhelming as it can be beautifully awesome.

Every Saturday at noon, the tsunami sirens are tested on Maui. As the tourists play, they pause a moment to wonder at the wailing noise, and then return to frolic in the ocean waves shaped like minitsunamis. But the sirens are a bitter reminder to the ka-

maainas, or "residents of Maui," that the chaos of life necessarily includes crisis and celebration, pleasure and pain.

The Gaia Hypothesis

As I write this chapter, I am surrounded by an endless array of indescribably bright colors and a lush green lawn contrasted against the dark blue sky. My landscape is back, but I am filled with an overpowering sense of the chaos that continues to create this paradise even as I write.

The tenth sacred secret of science is embodied in what is called the "Gaia hypothesis." Based on the "mother earth" of Greek mythology, this term was coined by author James Lovelock to explain his chaotic "daisy world" of self-sustaining processes and dynamic feedback.[6]

Greek mythology suggests that the earth is a goddess (Gaia) who imposes ultimate—although sometimes elusive—order amid the dynamic changes always taking place. The Gaia hypothesis suggests that the conditions for life spring from a self-sustaining, ever-changing feedback system: Order gives rise to disorder (entropy), which results in new order (neguentropy), which guarantees more disorder, and on and on forever.

Ilya Prigogine's theory of dissipative structures described in chapter 9 suggests that the falling apart of systems is one way that order is achieved. Dissipation, then, actually may be seen as the energy of coherence and as the spark of the Bose-Einstein condensate. The Gaia hypothesis is chaos theory's way of describing the earthly perturbations of divine dissipation that result in chaotic order.

The Gaia hypothesis explains how tidal waves can kill the native islanders who also find large schools of fish to feed their families from the same waters that drown them. The Gaia hypothesis helps us reconcile and explain how Heavenly Hana sprang from such a chaotic history and how my oleander plants, like life itself, can be both beautiful and lethal.

The Birth of Chaology

Meteorologist Edward Lorenz discovered, by coincidence, that the smallest variation in a set of numbers representing weather patterns can ultimately produce the ordered chaos of storms and tornadoes. In 1961, Lorenz made one slight change in how he ran the meteorology program on his computer. He simply started in the middle of the program rather than at the beginning and then let the computer run. That one small change created a wildly different hypothetical set of climatic conditions.

Like any good miracle maker, this founder of chaos theory refused to ignore this computer coincidence. He knew that his computer had not "gone wrong," but that something had "gone right" in an entirely new way. After seeing how a small variance of disorder resulted in an entirely new form of chaotic order, he made the miracle of an entirely new science called "chaos theory" or "chaology."

The Maharishi and the Butterfly

Lorenz's discovery of the impact of a small variation on the overall climate is now sometimes called the "Butterfly Effect."[7] Lorenz showed that, as James Gleick writes, "a butterfly stirring the air today in Peking can transform storm systems next month in New York."[8] Similarly one tiny DNA or genetic cross-link among millions of links in the cells in our bodies may produce cancer cells and a pattern of illness half a lifetime later. One cause of cancer is chaos, and I suggest that the ultimate "cure" for cancer will be found in the discovery of the order beneath its malignant chaos.

I have a brightly colored poster hanging in my college office. At first glance, students and visitors cannot tell what the poster is about. Closer examination reveals photographs of each letter of the alphabet made from patterns taken from the random array of colors on the wings of butterflies. This similarity between our alphabet and the patterns on the wings of butterflies is a coincidence of nature, but Kiell Sandved, a lecturer at the Smithsonian, has found three such "alphabetic coincidences" in more than 100,000 pairs of butterfly wings.[9] I use the poster to remind myself and my students that, if we look hard enough, we can find coincidental order anywhere and everywhere.

If small variations can produce major pattern changes, then small changes in our own consciousness might have profound effects on the order of the world. I have mentioned that on August 8, 1988, several followers of the Maharishi Mahesh Yogi, the founder of transcendental meditation, and other groups came to Haleakala to use their uncommon consciousness to help move the world toward more harmony. The assumption underlying their efforts is that a small, quantum leap of consciousness energy in each person could alter the entire energy field of the earth and all of its people. Believers in this effect gathered all over the world at "power points" where nature seemed to exert an exceptionally powerful energy. As I have pointed out, my magic mountain, Haleakala, is the most powerful of these places.

The Maharishi suggested that if only 1 percent of the earth's population entered into an uncommon consciousness—a spiritual awareness of our oneness and nonlocality—the other 99 percent of the population would be affected. Is it possible that the uncommon consciousness achieved on 8/8/88 helped to tear down the wall between East and West Germany and to promote the spread of democracy throughout Europe? Like butterfly wings, this uncommon consciousness on the part of a few could result in new vibrations that could change the spiritual climate of the world. The Maharishi Effect[10] is similar to the physics of coherence explained by the Bose-Einstein condensate theory: One small step toward an uncommon consciousness causes major leaps for personkind.

Sociologist Garland Landrith studied the Maharishi Effect and found that, in those U.S. cities where at least 1 percent of the population practiced "uncommon consciousness" (in this case, transcendental meditation), the crime rate was significantly lowered.[11] The Landrith studies have been replicated several times with the same results.

At the 1981 American Psychological Association convention in Los Angeles, I heard psychologist Michael Dillbeck present a paper in which he described his study of whether there was a direct cause-and-effect relationship between a small but powerful change in consciousness and the crime rate in the cities where such changes took place.[12] Through complex mathematical experimental design, he showed that the crime rate in the transcendental meditation cities was reduced as a *direct* result of the consciousness change in the 1 percent of the population, thus affecting the other 99 percent.

Traffic movement at rush hour, immune system function, blood chemistry, heart rhythms, and cell division all have been proven to contain a chaotic order emerging from small fluctuations. The messes and miracles in our own lives are small events in the overall scheme of things, but they are ultimately as powerful as a butterfly's wings or a Maharishi's meditation.

Jagged Geometry and Fractal Art

Mathematician Benoit Mandelbrot worked as a researcher for the International Business Machines Corporation in the early 1960s. He, along with Edward Lorenz, Douglas Hofstadter, Bruce Stewart, Roderick Jensen, and the leading spokesman for the new chaology, Joseph Ford, have proved that, as Ford writes, chaos exists as "dynamics freed at last from the shackles of order and predictability . . . a cornucopia of opportunity."[13]

Mandelbrot applied his mathematics to several different domains of reality. Refusing to limit himself to one view of the order of things, Mandelbrot was willing to seek meaning and pattern in what appeared to be random coincidence. As a result, he was able to extend the principles of chaology to other domains of science such as economics and politics.

Mandelbrot used mathematical systems to measure fractional, nonlinear, irregular things such as coastlines and the edges of snowflakes. Unlike the smooth and perfect curves drawn by students plotting linear equations, nonlinear solutions to problems show turbulence, breaks, and explosions of discontinuity.[14]

One day, as Mandlebrot was casually thumbing through his son's Latin dictionary, by coincidence he came across the Latin word *fractus*, which means "to break." Mandelbrot gave meaning to this coincidence. He named the "rougher" but beautifully complex dimensions and patterns he was dealing with in his mathematics "fractals." Images of these fractals are now the basis of scientific work all over the world.

Using a special kit that her parents had bought for her (called a Spirograph), Patsy could draw nonlinear, fractional figures by using a plastic template and a pencil. The images were the beautiful swirls and curves of linear geometry, but Patsy loved to make the slightest alteration to "mess the thing up so it looks more real." By making one little change, the patterns became beautifully turbulent and disordered. "I like it this way better," Patsy said. Patsy's

pictures were a "jagged geometry" of chaos. When such pictures
are drawn by computers, magnificently artistic images and patterns dance across the screen. Computer hobbyists enjoy playing
with these pictures of chaos.

Chaos on the Nile

The river that many historians feel to be the cradle of civilization,
the Nile, varies tremendously in its depth. The Egyptians kept
careful records of what at first appear to be the totally random
inexplicable flooding and extremely low river levels. By examining
the millennia of Nile River records using his "fractal" system,
Mandelbrot found an ordered chaos that he summarized in two
"effects" that he called the Noah and Joseph effects.[15]

According to Mandelbrot, the Noah effect, like the biblical
Flood, represented the *spontaneous discontinuity*, or chaotic patterns, of changes in the world. Changes may not take place for long
periods of time, but then as if by a quantum leap, a chaotic coincidence occurs and a flood or perhaps a tsunami results. Mandelbrot
extended this example to economics, where price and interest
changes do not, in fact, change smoothly and gradually as many
economists predict. Instead, they occur as suddenly as computers
can send messages. The stock market is more likely to crash than
to deteriorate slowly, for example.

In contrast, the Joseph effect stood for the opposite factors of
continuity and *persistence*. The biblical legend of a historical pattern
of seven years of plenty and seven years of famine represents the
periodicity of life, just as the Nile would eventually crest even after
years of drought. The more things stay the same, the more the
same they seem to become—as persons living through droughts
feel that their drought has lasted and will last forever. In the overall
nature of chaos, however, sameness is the best predictor of change,
for the tenth secret of science teaches that just when things seem
stable, something will "mess them up"; and when things seem
totally helter-skelter, they will eventually settle down for a while.
In this sense, sameness predicts change and change is the best
predictor of sameness.

When we are experiencing the Noah effect, we may feel as if we
are being drowned by problem after problem, but in the ultimate

chaotic order, sameness and persistence will occur. We may feel that we are bored and stuck in sameness, but that is only because we do not see the subtle oscillations that are occurring to create constant change on the universal level.

Why Do Miracles Seem So Sudden

To visit Hana now and see the lovely town nestled safely in the quiet, rolling bay would not give anyone but people like my *kahuna* gardener Pete the slightest hint of the threat of a tidal wave. Similarly, when we are seriously ill, it's easy to lose sight of the fact that no matter how long and how badly we suffer, things do change. Some small variation takes place, and a flood of healing can occur. Conversely, when things seem very good for us, we can be sure that we will eventually experience crises in our life. We can live our life in dread of future problems, or we can accept the fact that we could not exist if we were not, like all of the cosmos, in the process of constant change and remember that the definition of the word *dread* is not only "fear and apprehension" but also "deep awe and reverence."[16] The miracle makers whom I studied were characterized by their awe for living much more than by their terror of change and challenge.

The crumbling of the Berlin Wall in late 1989, less than a year after the 8/8/88 consciousness convergence exercise described earlier in this chapter, and the accompanying spread of democracy all over the world seems to have taken place almost all at once. We wonder how, after so many years of oppression, freedom can so spontaneously break out all over the world. Chaology might explain that some comparatively small change (the 8/8/88 meetings?) is now playing itself out. And just when things seem to be stabilizing in one direction, war begins in the Middle East. Peace and conflict may appear to emerge suddenly, but they are the result of the impact of small changes resulting in major consequences. All miracles seem sudden, but they are formed by the subtle changes that we ourselves make in our view of life. Until our political leaders understand miracle making, they will continue to obstruct the orderly flow through chaos by trying to have their own wills be done rather than helping all of us discover and pray for Thy will so that all of us together can make the miracle of peace.

Where the Whales Win

The humpback whale is about fifty feet long and weighs more than forty tons. These magnificent creatures congregate in the warm Maui waters every year to give birth to their little 2,000-pound babies.[17] While visiting Maui, the whales do not eat. They parent and play as the screams of delighted tourists spotting a humpback whale's huge dorsal fin are heard from December through March. The splash of the humpback's fifteen-foot flipper slapping the water in a statement of territoriality can be heard echoing for miles off the slopes of Haleakala and the west Maui mountains.

The whales' favorite playground is just off the shore of Lahina on Maui. There, they seem to be calling the tourists out to play. It seems that they are celebrating their victory over the whalers who killed thousands of their ancestors swimming in these same waters, decimating their numbers from the 200,000 alive at the turn of the century to the 7,000 or so that now survive. Centuries of chaotic slaughter have been replaced by a rush of tourists in awe of whale's grandeur.

Today, visitors go out in small boats to photograph rather than harpoon these great animals. The boats full of tourists toss helplessly, nearly capsizing as the ocean swells have their way. Cameras fly into the water and everyone hangs on for dear life as they try to catch a glimpse of the humpbacks playing with their young.

When whalers walked the narrow streets of old Lahina town, the sailors were the masters. To them, it must have seemed that this was a way of life that would last forever. They chased, harassed, and killed the whales, and then celebrated their killing by reveling in the warm and healthy climate and people of Lahina. Everything seemed stable and predictable and "the way it would always be." But it was not "the way it is."

Eventually, chaos changes everything and anything. Small things are always happening that will bring major changes. Molecular discoveries resulted in new approaches to energy and fuel, so the demand for whale oil decreased sharply. Invisible viruses brought by the sailors began to kill the native Hawaiians. The sea captains' anger at the interference of the missionaries in their lustful pursuits resulted in sailors sneaking ashore at night to plant tiny larva in the ponds near the missionaries' homes, so that a paradise free of blood-sucking insects then had its first mosquitoes. Small changes had chaotic results, and a paradise was lost.

Now, the tourists walk in Lahina with T-shirts that are printed with "I'm having a whale of a time." Massive hotels line the beaches. Another celebration of a different life of excess is underway. Yet small changes are again taking place amid the new order. Overdevelopment and pollution are planting the seeds of another chaos in paradise.

The Whales' Chant

Humpback whales communicate through their singing. It is a grunting, shrieking, mournful sound. I listened to tapes of the whales playing in the waters near my Maui home when I lay in pain, and the whales' crooning soothed me. Each whale sings exactly the same song, which lasts about twenty minutes and is repeated over and over again much like an ancient Hawaiian chant. The whales' song reverberates through Maui when the whales come, echoing back and forth between the west or head-shaped mountains and the east or heart-shaped mountains of Maui.

Yet there is a chaos in the humpback whales' chant. Their songs change every year. They are similar in form to the construction of a complex symphonic work, yet every whale learns the new tunes. The whales come back each year with last year's songs and then compose new melodies. Their notes become so forceful that they can be heard above and below the water for miles. The bass notes carry underwater for more than 100 miles, and when we swim under the water, we can feel the vibrations of the whales' resonating deep within our chests. It is likely that it was whale songs vibrating through the wooden decks of the old ships that were the mournful songs of the Sirens of Greek mythology who lured whale-killing sailors to their own deaths.

I have heard the whales' new song every year, and like most people who listen to the whales singing, I can feel my shared consciousness with them. Scientists have studied the humpback whale's new yearly songs for decades and have yet to find the pattern in the chaos. I suspect that their chaos *is* their pattern.

In his novel *Moby Dick*, Herman Melville wrote, "The classification of the constituents of a chaos, nothing less here is essayed."

We and all that we do and feel are the constituents of chaos. That makes the whales and us demi-gods in the tradition of Maui.

Psychologist Abraham Maslow writes of the Jonah complex, or our fear of becoming all that we can be and of realizing our potential as human beings.[18] Jonah became entrapped inside a whale (actually the Bible says it was a large fish and not a whale) partly because he failed to see his personal strength and power to be more than what he was. Maslow called this avoidance of our godlike capacity an "escape from greatness" and wrote, "If we deliberately set out to be less than we are capable, we'll be unhappy for the rest of our lives."[19] Making miracles is our potential. To do less is to be swallowed up by our fear of chaos rather than our search for meaning within it.

"Why Me?" and Chaos

My wife and I were flying to Rome where I was scheduled to give one of my first post-illness lectures on the making of miracles. It was only weeks since I had been in intensive care, dying. My bone marrow transplant was only months old, yet here I was, going to Europe! I was discussing this miracle with my wife and was indirectly asking the "Why me?" question by saying, "I can't believe this happened to me!" The tsunami of my illness had passed, and it seemed like we were in heaven.

Our meal of Italian steak had just been served, and at just that moment, the flight attendant leaned over and asked in broken English, "Did you want more marrow?"

I could not believe my ears. I turned to my wife, who also seemed startled. "What?" she said. "What do you mean?"

The flight attendant gestured to a saucer he was holding and said, "Would you like more marrow sauce on your steak?"

"No thank you," said my wife quietly. We did not say a word to one another as we considered what had just happened. "Just another coincidence in our chaotic life," said my wife as she tucked the menu away as proof of yet another significant coincidence in our life.

Chaology's answer to "Why me?" is that *we* are all fractals, and we are all a part of the system of chaotic order. We may feel that our chaos is personal, but it is pervasive and natural to our existence.

Only on the local level of reality does our suffering seem to be solo. As a part of the cosmic whole, we are all a part of a much more complex symphony of life.

"Why Now?" and a Terrible Coincidence

As our flight to Rome continued and the flight attendants were removing our trays, an announcement came over the public address system. Something was said in Italian, and half of the passengers on the plane gasped, shuffled nervously, and then laughed. We waited eagerly for the English translation.

"I'm so sorry to have to tell you that something terrible has happened," said the head flight attendant. Now, the other half of the passengers gasped. "They forgot to load our plane with the movie for today's flight. We will not have a movie today."

In that short and probably twelve-second moment, we had gone from a feeling of impending air disaster to the minor inconvenience of a missed movie. In the same plane at almost the same time, one-half of the passengers had lived momentarily in terror while the other half had been calm in their sense of sameness. This "terrible coincidence" seemed to reveal chaology's answer to the "Why now?" question: Time, like everything in the universe, is chaotic. We experience moments of terror and moments of peacefulness. When these moments occur is a matter of chaotic order, not the flow of linear time.

"Now What?" and Surviving a Lightning Strike

I was sitting next to a flight attendant on a small plane headed for Traverse City, Michigan. I was still thinking about the woman who had been assigned that seat so many times that day and about the coincidence of my gate number matching her seat number. As is often the case in early summer in Michigan, thunderstorms were in the area, but our flight was proceeding smoothly.

Suddenly, there was a loud crack. The entire cabin of the plane turned a bright and blinding white, and a fog of smoke rose from just beside my seat. "My God," said the flight attendant. "That hit right at your feet. We've been struck by lightning."

With measured calm, the captain announced that we had indeed suffered a strong lightning strike, but that everything on the plane seemed to be in working order. "I can't tell if the landing gear or electrical landing controls will work until we are ready to land." he added, "but I don't expect any problems." He then said that we had to fly back to Detroit where "they have better emergency equipment."

Everyone sat in silence as we flew back through the same storm that had caused the lightning to hit us. As the plane lurched and jumped through the turbulence of the storm, the circumstances seemed to elicit among the passengers just the right response to the question of "Now what?" during times of crisis and chaos. We did and said nothing. It is the same warning that is painted above the explode button of the ejection seat on fighter jets. "First, do nothing," says the sign. If we can first do nothing and then seize the moment, we can more fully experience and learn from chaos rather than resist and panic.

"Just my luck," I said to the tense flight attendant.

"You mean things haven't been going well for you lately?" she asked. "Maybe you're the reason we got struck by lightning" she joked and moved away from me. "That lightning bolt hit right at your feet. See the burn marks?" I looked down and saw a streak of black running from the back of my seat toward my feet. No other place on the plane showed evidence of the hit.

"No, I mean, just my luck. I've been making miracles like crazy," I said. "You folks are lucky I'm on this plane."

The flight attendant laughed and said, "You know, being a flight attendant or a pilot is sort of like life in general. Hours of boredom and five minutes of panic. That's just the way it is." I thought, "She's just summarized chaos theory in one eight-word sentence."

"So What?" and the Clues of Chaos

As we heard the strong thud of the landing gear locking into place, a collective groan of relief spread throughout the plane. The pilot's voice was heard over the public address system once again. "Everything is fine, ladies and gentlemen. Nature just reached out and touched someone, and that someone was us. In a moment, your flight attendant, Patsy, will have some gate information for you."

I had sat next to Patsy throughout the flight, and I probably could have guessed her name. I had felt her insight, energy, and depth of feeling. Her name fit well.

As we taxied toward the terminal, the flight attendant said, "We will be arriving at gate . . ." and then there was a pause. I could see her trying to attach a strap that held a tray, and she was distracted from the paper in front of her. I wondered if we would return to gate 7A. We did not.

"We'll be arriving at gate eight at just about eight P.M.," she said, looking directly at me and then resuming her work. I wanted to tell everyone on that plane about yet another meaningful coincidence.

The "So what?" question is answered by chaology through the promise and meaning chaos holds for us. If we are alert to the coincidences in our lives, we will see the clues that there is always an ultimate order. If we have faith in our nonlocality and oneness rather than a fear of running out of time on our predestined march to the end of "me" or of those we love, we learn that the meaning in life's chaos will always be revealed to us. We can be free to celebrate our human spirit even at the bad times in our lives when we apply Patsy's principle that "it's just the way it is."

A Cosmic Thumbprint

We had been on a very small plane, and as we descended the narrow steps to the tarmac, we all could look back at the side of the fuselage where the lightning had struck. Even though there was a light rain falling and the possibility of more lightning, no one went into the terminal. The pilot, copilot, and Patsy the flight attendant came to look. What we saw burned into the side of the plane was a miracle.

Along the right side of the fuselage, starting near the window near my seat and ending near the tail, was a long, swirling, deep black pattern. One little girl said, "Mamma, look what God did. He made a big smudge on the side of our airplane." We all looked more closely as we tentatively touched the warm black line. It was inscribed into the metal as if scorched there by a torch. There was still an odor of burned metal.

As we walked away from the plane, we kept looking back at the mark. From a different and farther view, the smudge was really a pattern of swirls that circled from the window by my seat to about ten windows back. It was a perfect set of swirls. It was an image of a fractal. It was a long series of intertwined number eights lying on their side in a chain of joined infinity signs. I felt like cheering, but instead I started to cry.

"Getting wet?" asked Patsy as she looked at my wet cheeks. "Or are you crying?" I couldn't answer. "You should be glad we're walking into the terminal instead of being terminal. Everything's in order now. We're all fine." She'll never know why, but I gave her a hug before walking down the hall.

As I confront the miracle of my cure from cancer and recovery from my bone marrow transplant, I face the most severe challenge of my entire ordeal. Every twitch, pain, or ache still frightens me. "Is it coming back?" I wonder. "Did the miracle really happen?"

Adjusting to wellness and accepting chaos as health is not easy. It is as difficult as coping with illness. Like Captain Ahab and his obsession with the white whale Moby Dick, I felt tied to my crisis and almost consumed by it. If I could not free myself from the bonds of my fear and obsession, I would drown.

There is constant disbelief and even resentment on the part of some people who do not understand that miracles can be made. There is doubt by former employers, companies who would hire me to lecture, and even publishers who could not believe that I am writing, lecturing, and touring again.

Making miracles is the easy part, for you have read about the new scientific principles that guide the way. The difficult part for all of us is to find the meaning in the miracle. I believe the meaning is that there is a lovely, sacred chaos to the development of our soul. Every coincidence hints at it. Every miracle we make proves it. We make our miracles through our prayers, our creativity, our sacred time, our connection to one another, our faith, and most of all, through our celebration of life's miraculous "way" of teaching us about the evolution of our human spirit.

NOTES

1. Steven Weinberg, *The First Three Minutes* (New York: Basic Books, 1976).
2. Ed Regis, *Who's Got Einstein's Office* (Reading, MA: Addison-Wesley, 1987).

3. James Gleick, *Chaos: Making a New Science* (New York: Penguin Books, 1987), 314.

4. Quoted in *Ibid.*, 314.

5. *Ibid.*, 279.

6. This hypothesis and its relationship to the order beneath chaos is found in John E. Lovelock and described in *Ibid.*, 279. See also James E. Lovelock, *Gaia: A New Look at Life on Earth* (Oxford, UK: Oxford University Press, 1979).

7. Edward Lorenz first described the "Butterfly Effect" in a paper he titled "Predictability: Does the Flap of a Butterfly's Wings in Brazil Set Off a Tornado in Texas," presented at the annual meeting of the American Association for the Advancement of Science in Washington, DC, Dec. 29, 1979.

8. *Ibid.*, 8.

9. Kiell Sandved noticed, by coincidence, that there was a perfect letter *F* in a butterfly wing he saw fifteen years ago. His creativity and search for more coincidences and an order in chaos resulted in beautiful posters, *Sandved and Coleman Photo*, Fairfax, VA

10. Elaine Aron and Arthur Aron, *The Maharishi Effect: A Revolution Through Meditation* (Walpole, NH: Stillpoint, 1986).

11. C. Borland and Garland Landrith, "Improved Quality of City Life Through the Transcendental Meditation Program: Decreased Crime Rate," in *Scientific Research of the Transcendental Meditation and TM-Siddhi Program: Collected Papers*, vol. 1 (Livingston Manor, NY: Maharishi International University Press, 1973).

12. Michael C. Dillbeck, "Social Field Effects in Crime Prevention," paper presented at the annual convention of the American Psychological Association, Los Angeles, 1981; and Michael C. Dillbeck, G. S. Landrith, C. Polanzi, and S. R. Baker, "The Transcendental Mediation Program and Crime Rate Change: A Causal Analysis," in *Scientific Research of the Transcendental Meditation and TM-Siddhi Program: Collected Papers*, vol. 4 (Livingston Manor, NY: Maharishi International University Press, 1973).

13. Quoted in Gleick, *Chaos*, 306.

14. For an excellent introduction to "chaotic wholeness," see J. Briggs and D. Peat, *Turbulent Mirror* (New York: Harper & Row, 1989).

15. Benoit Mandelbrot, *The Fractal Geometry of Nature* (New York: W. H. Freeman, 1977). This is a highly technical, encyclopedic work, but it is one of the most comprehensive expositions on the occurrence of fractals of "ordered chaos patterns" occurring throughout nature.

16. *The American College Dictionary* (New York: Random House, 1960), 366.

17. An excellent and brief review of some of the legends and science of Maui is found in J. D. Bisignani, *Maui Handbook* (Chico, CA: Moon Publication, 1988).

18. The evolution of Abraham Maslow's thinking about the Jonah complex is traced in Edward Hoffman, *The Right to Be Human: The Biography of Abraham Maslow* (Los Angeles: Tarcher, 1988), 298. In the biblical tale, Jonah feared his own greatness, and our almost willful failure to develop to our full human potential (to make miracles?) was described much earlier by historian Frank Manuel, *Shapes of Philosophical History* (Stanford, CA: Stanford University Press, 1965).

19. Hoffman, *The Right to Be Human*, 298.

PEARSALL'S PROPAEDEUTICS

A Miracle Maker's Manual

Nobody gets "their" way. We all get "the" way.
—PATSY

The word *propaedeutic* refers to "the study of the basic and organizing principles or rules of a field of science or art." I began using the word in my lectures more than twenty years ago to refer to the importance of understanding the fundamentals of all of the sciences before attempting to learn the specifics of one science. My students found *propaedeutics* to be an unusual-sounding word, and I hoped that this strangeness would help them remember two things—the same two points that I have emphasized throughout this book.

First, there are more basic rules of the universe than can be discovered by the processes of our see-and-touch world. These rules come from substantiated findings of a new science that stretches the limits of our thinking, awareness, and spirituality. The beautiful simplicity and wide applicability of these remarkable ways of understanding the cosmos can help us find a new meaning to the chaos in our lives.

Second, miracles can be made using these basic principles. The four C's of the cycle of life—coincidence, crisis, cure, and chaos—

are all clues to the way in which science and religion coalesce in the making of miracles. I have developed "ten commandments" for miracle making based on these clues.

I hope you will find my "miracle maker's manual" helpful in fashioning your own miracles. Like the demi-god Maui, we can learn to pull the meaning of life from the sea of chaos and make our own sacred time. In Hawaiian, I wish you what the *kahunas* chanted from the top of Haleakala: *Ka maluhia o ka i*, or "the ultimate peace of your soul."

Pearsall's Propaedeutics

1. We are free from the limits of linear, local space and time. Thoughts, feelings, and love can have their effect all at once, anywhere, at any time. The scientific principle of *nonlocality* proves the reality of instantaneous action. Miracles can be made suddenly and can have their effects everywhere all at once. *Be Reverent of your free, ubiquitous, and common spirit.*

2. We create our world by what, how, and when we choose to interpret the events in our lives. The act of observing is the act of creating. The scientific principle of *observer participancy* proves that observers are necessary to bring the world into being. We create our miracles using a vision beyond our eyesight—miracles form through our "soul sight." *Be cognizant of the transformative power of your perceptions.*

3. We live in a universe of parallels. There is always an opposite side to every event, feeling, fear, and hope. The *complementarity principle* proves that we are energy and mass, wave and particle, lumps and jumps; we are quantum stuff in progress. Each way of knowing something proves the existence of another "way." Miracles are made when we remember that "one and one makes One." *Be reflective about the duality of all persons, things, and events.*

4. We can never be certain of anything. The scientific *principle of uncertainty* proves that the more we know of one side or one aspect of something, the less we know of its other side. We should never "rest assured." The more our knowledge, the greater our ignorance. Miracles result from our recognition that even the worst news is only a short story; the whole

plot is an unfolding mystery. *Be humble in your perpetual uncertainty.*

5. We are not an isolated mind and consciousness. The scientific *principle of oneness* proves that miracles are created from our efforts to acknowledge, be aware of, and think as one mind. All miracles are group efforts. *Be prayerful as your ultimate source of miracle-making power.*

6. There is more than one reality. The scientific *principle of many realms of reality* proves that there are several domains of reality and that each realm has its own rules and ways of explaining the universe. We do not have to "face reality." We make miracles by embracing *all* of the realities. *Be creative in constructing your own reality and in your reading of coincidences.*

7. Because we decide how we will move through our world, time travel is possible. The scientific *principle of simultaneity* proves that it is possible on some levels of reality to "cosmically commute" at superluminal, or faster than light, speeds. Miracles are made when we create sacred time—reverence for "moments"—and not the profane time of "one hurried day at a time." *Carpe momentum* is the orientation of the miracle maker. *Be patient and make all of your time sacred.*

8. We are surrounded by fields of energy that determine our development. The scientific *principle of vibrational energy* proves that our bodies, even when they are damaged or diseased, are wonderful vessels for the temporary and local organizing of the energy of our spirits. Miracles are made when we free ourselves from the idea that "we are our bodies." *Be connected with the loving energy around you.*

9. We are constantly falling apart, and that is how we eventually get it all together. The scientific *principle of neguentropy* and the Laws of Thermodynamics prove that the turmoil and commotion in our lives are necessary and natural processes for reorganization of the spirit. A miracle is made by *using* rather than *fearing* our moments of disaster. *Be hopeful of a miracle.*

10. Existence causes chaos, and chaos is the ultimate cause of ever-evolving order. The scientific findings of *chaology* prove that the very point of our existence is the chaos we create by the agitation of our presence in the universe. The coinci-

dences, crises, cures, and chaos of our daily lives prove our disruptive but magnificent cosmic influence. We make the ultimate miracle when we discover the meaning of life's disorder: that, like the violent tsunamis and the volcanoes that formed the paradise of Maui, existence is a beautiful chaos. *Be joyful that miracles can be made by any and all of us.*

The visits of the humpback whales to Maui always remind me that we become miracle makers amid chaos by freeing ourselves from our Ahab complex. Like Ahab in Herman Melville's *Moby Dick*, we tend to become obsessed with the fears and ambitions of our see-and-touch, cause-and-effect world. Like Ahab, if we become trapped in these preoccupations, we eventually drown in the wreckage of our strivings and yearnings.

We take our first steps on the path from local pain to cosmic joy when our faith, supported by science, frees us to find an uncommon consciousness. When we take these first tentative steps along the way to making miracles, we accept Thoreau's challenge to "live deep and suck out all the marrow of life," and to "put to route" all that is not a full and rich chaotic life, so that we do not, when we come to die, discover that we have not lived.

BIBLIOGRAPHY

For further information on bone marrow transplant, obtain a free booklet titled *Friends Helping Friends: A Bone Marrow Transplant Resource Guide* by calling (800) 825–2536. To talk personally with someone who has received a bone marrow transplant or a family member of a patient, call this same number. Remember, the feelings and opinions expressed will be based on that individual's own experience and do *not* constitute medical advice. Each case is unique, so see your doctor for referral for information regarding your own individual situation.

Abell, O., and Singer, B., eds. *Science and the Paranormal: Probing the Existence of the Supernatural.* New York: Charles Scribner's Sons, 1981.

Ackerman, Diane. *A Natural History of the Senses.* New York: Random House, 1990.

American College Dictionary. New York: Random House, 1960.

Aristotle. *Basic Works,* ed. Richard McKeon. New York: Random House, 1941.

Aron, E., and Aron, A. *The Maharishi Effect: A Revolution Through Meditation.* Walpole, NH: Stillpoint Publishing, 1986.

Bateson, M. C. "The Revenge of the Good Fairy." *Whole Earth Review* 55 (Summer 1987): 34–48.

Bisignani, J. D. *Maui Handbook.* Chico, CA: Moon Publications, 1988.

Borland, C., and Landrith, G. *Improved Quality of City Life Through the Transcendental Meditation and TM-Siddhi Program: Collected Papers,* vol. 1. Livingston Manor, NY: Maharishi International University Press, 1973.

Briggs, J., and Peat, F. "David Bohm's Looking-Glass Map," in *Looking Glass Universe: The Emerging Science of Wholeness.* New York: Simon & Schuster, 1984.

Briggs, J., and Peat, F. *Turbulent Mirror.* New York: Harper & Row, 1989.

Buber, M. *I and Thou.* Edinburgh, UK: T. & T. Clark, 1937.

Bucke, R. *Cosmic Consciousness.* New York: E. P. Dutton, 1969.

Bucke, W. "From Self to Cosmic Consciousness," in *The Highest State of Consciousness,* ed. J. White, Garden City, NY: Doubleday, 1972.

Burr, H. S. *The Fields of Life.* New York: Ballantine Books, 1972.

Byrd, R. C. "Positive Therapeutic Effects of Intercessory Prayer in a Coronary Care Unit Population." *Southern Medical Journal* 81, no. 7 (1988), 36–78.

Cassirer, E. *The Philosophy of the Enlightenment.* Princeton, NJ: Princeton University Press, 1951.

Cavendish, R., ed. *Encyclopedia of the Unexplained: Magic, Occultism, and Parapsychology.* New York: Penguin Books, 1989.

Combs, A., and Holland, M. *Synchronicity: Science, Myth, and the Trickster.* New York: Paragon House, 1990.

Csikszentmihalyi, M. *Flow: The Psychology of Optimal Experience.* New York: HarperCollins, 1990.

Darwin, Charles. *The Expression of the Emotions in Man and Animals.* London: Longmans, 1872.

Darwin, Charles. *On the Origin of Species by Means of Natural Selection, or the Preservation of Favoured Races in the Struggle for Life.* 1959.

Davies, P. *God and the New Physics.* New York: Simon & Schuster, 1983.

de Chardin, P. Teilhard. *The Phenomenon of Man.* New York: Harper & Row, 1959.

Demitrescu, I. "Life Energy Patterns Visible Via New Techniques." *Brain/ Mind Bulletin* 7, no. 14 (1982).

Dienstbier, R. "Arousal and Physiological Toughness: Implications for Mental and Physical Health." *Psychological Review* 96, no. 1 (1989): 84–100.

Dillbeck, M. C. "Social Field Effects in Crime Prevention." Paper presented at the Annual Convention of the American Psychological Association, Los Angeles, 1981.

Dillbeck, M. C., Landrith, G. S., Polanzi, C., and Baker, S. R. "The Transcendental Meditation Program and Crime Rate Change: A Causal

Analysis." In *Scientific Research of the Transcendental Meditation and TM-Siddhi Program: Collected Papers*, vol. 4. Livingston Manor, NY: Maharishi International University Press, 1973.

Dossey, L. *Space, Time, and Medicine*. Boulder: Shambhala, 1982.

Dossey, L. *Recovering the Soul: A Scientific and Spiritual Search*. New York: Bantam Books, 1989.

Eidson, W. W., Faust, D. L., Kyler, H. J., Pehek, J. O., and Poock, G. K. "Kirlian Photography." *Proceedings of the Insititue of Electrical and Electronic Engineers Conference*. Boston, 1978.

Eliade, M. *The Sacred and the Profane*. New York: Harcourt Brace and World, 1959.

Eliade, M. *Shamanism*. Princeton, NJ: Princeton University Press, 1964.

Eliade, M. *Patterns in Comparative Religion*. New York: New American Library, 1974.

Fink, John M. *Third Opinion*. New York: Avery Publishing Group, 1988.

Finkelstein, D. "A Theory of the Vacuum," in *Philosophy of the Vacuum*, ed. S. Saunders. Oxford, UK: Oxford University Press, 1989.

Frolich, H. "Coherent Excitations in Active Biological Systems," in *Modern Bioelectrochemistry*, ed. F. Gutman and H. Keyzer. New York: Plenum, 1986.

Gallagher, P. "Over Easy: A Cultural Anthropologist's Near-Death Experience." *Abiosis* 2, no. 2 (1982).

Gerard, R. "Units and Concepts of Biology." *Science* 125 (1957).

Gerber, R. *Vibrational Medicine: New Choices for Healing Ourselves*. Santa Fe: Bear Company, 1988.

"Ghost Effect." *IKRA Communications* (June 1978).

Gleick, J. *Chaos: Making a New Science*. New York: Penguin Books, 1987.

Goleman, D. *Vital Lies, Simple Truths*. New York: Simon & Schuster, 1985.

Hadamard, J. *The Psychology of Invention in the Mathematical Field*. Princeton, NJ: Princeton University Press, 1945.

Hardie, A., Harvie, R., and Koestler, A. *The Challenge of Chance*. London: Hutchinson, 1973.

Harton, J. J. "An Investigation on the Influence of Success and Failure on the Estimation of Time." *Journal of General Psychology* 21 (1938): 51–62.

Hawking, S. *A Brief History of Time*. New York: Bantam Books, 1988.

Hay, Louise L. *You Can Heal Yourself*. Santa Monica, CA: Louise May Publisher, 1984.

Hayward, J. W. *Perceiving Ordinary Magic*. Boulder, CO: Shambhala, 1984.

Hayward, J. *Shifting Worlds, Changing Minds: Where the Sciences and Buddhism Meet*. Boston: Shambhala, 1987.

Heinberg, R. *Memories and Visions of Paradise: Exploring the Universal Myth of a Lost Golden Age*. Los Angeles: Jeremy P. Tarcher, 1989.

Heisenberg, W. *Physics and Beyond*. New York: Harper & Row, 1971.

Herbert, N. *Quantum Reality*. New York: Anchor Books, 1987.

Hey, T., and Walters, P. *The Quantum Universe*. Cambridge, UK: Cambridge University Press, 1989.

Hoffman, Enid. *Huna: A Beginner's Guide*. West Chester, PA: Whitford Press, 1981.

Hoffman, Eugene. *The Right to Be Human: The Biography of Abraham Maslow*. Los Angeles: Jeremy P. Tarcher, Inc., 1988.

Hoveyda, F. F. "The Image of Science in Our Society." *Bioscience Communications III* no. 3 (1977).

Hume, D. *Enquiry Concerning Human Understanding*, ed. L. A. S. Bigge. New York: Greenword Press, 1980.

Huxley, A. *The Perennial Philosophy*. New York: Harper & Row, 1944.

Hynek, J. A. "The Emerging Picture of the UFO Problem." *American Institute of Aeronautics and Astronautics* 75, no. 41 (1975).

Jackson, J. H. *Selected Writings*. London: Hodder and Stoughton, 1931.

Jantsch, E. *The Self-Organizing Universe*. New York: Pergamon, 1980.

Jung, C. *Analytical Psychology: Its Theory and Practice: The Tavistock Lectures*. New York: Random House, 1968.

Jung, C. "Synchronicity: An Acausal Connecting Principles," in *Collected Works*, vol. 8. Princeton, NJ: Princeton University Press, 1973.

Kammerer, P. *Das Gestex der Serie*. Stuttgart-Berlin: Deutsche Veriags-Ansalt, 1919.

Koestler, A. *The Roots of Coincidence*. New York: Random House, 1972.

Koestler, A. *The Case of the Midwife Toad*. New York: Random House, 1973.

Krippner, S., ed. *Energies of Consciousness*. New York: Gordon & Breach, 1975.

Krippner, S., and Rubin, D. *The Kirlian Aura*. New York: Anchor, 1974.

LeShan, L., and Marenau, H. *Einstein's Space and Van Gogh's Sky: Physical Reality and Beyond*. New York: Macmillan Publishing Co., 1982.

Locke, S., and Colligan, D. *The Healer Within*. New York: E. P. Dutton, 1986.

Long, M. F. *The Secret Science Behind Miracles*. Santa Monica, CA: DeVorss, 1948.

Lorenz, E. "Predictability: Does the Flap of a Butterfly's Wings in Brazil Set off a Tornado in Texas." Paper presented at the annual meeting of American Association for Advancement of Science in Washington, DC: Dec. 29, 1979.

Lovelock, J. E. *Gaia: A New Look at Life on Earth*. Oxford, UK: Oxford University Press, 1979.

MacLean, P. "On the Evolution of the Three Mentalities." In *New Dimensions in Psychiatry: A World View*, vol. 2, ed. S. Arieti and G. Chrzanowki. New York: John Wiley & Sons, 1977.

MacMillan, R. L., and Brown, K. W. G. "Cardiac Arrest Remembered." *The Canadian Medical Association Journal* 104 (1971).

Mallikarjun, S. "Kirlian Photography in Cancer Diagnosis." *Osteopathic Physician* 45, no. 5 (1978): 24–27.

Mandelbrot, B. *The Fractal Geometry of Nature*. New York: W. H. Freeman, 1977.

Mandell, A. J. "From Molecular Biological Simplification to More Realistic Central Nervous System Dynamics: An Opinion," in *Psychobiological Foundations of Clinical Psychiatry*. vol. 3, no. 2, ed. J. O. Cavenar et al. Philadelphia: J. B. Lippincott, 1985.

Manuel, F. *Shapes of Philosophical History*. Stanford, CA: Stanford University Press, 1965.

Maslow, A. *The Farther Reaches of Human Nature*. New York: Viking, 1971.

Masters, W., and Johnson, V. *Human Sexual Response*. Boston: Little, Brown, 1966.

Melzack, R., and Wall, P. "Pain Mechanisms: A New Theory." *Science* 150 (1965): 971–979.

Michener, J. A. *Hawaii*. New York: Ballantine Books, 1959.

Mindel, A. "Synchronicity, An Investigation of the Unitary Background Patterning Synchronous Phenomenon." *Dissertation Abstracts International* 37, no. 2 (1976).

Monod, J. *Chance and Necessity*. New York: Alfred A. Knopf, 1971.

Moody, R. *Reflections of Life after Life*. New York: Bantam Books, 1977.

Morowitz, H. *Energy Flow in Biology.* Woodridge, CT: Ox Bow Press, 1979.

Morowitz, H. *Cosmic Joy and Local Pain: Musing of a Mystic Scientist.* New York: Charles Scribner's Sons, 1987.

Morris, H. M. *The Troubled Waters of Evolution.* San Diego, CA: Creation-Life Publishers, 1975.

Moss, T. "Puzzles and Promises." *Osteopathic Physician* (1976).

Moss, T. *The Body Electric.* Los Angeles: J. P. Tarcher, Inc., 1979.

Murchie, G. *The Seven Mysteries of Life: An Exploration of Science and Philosophy.* Boston: Houghton Mifflin Co., 1978.

Newsweek. Oct. 22, 1990.

Nicolis, G., and Prigogine, I. *Self-Organization in Non-Equilibrium Systems* New York: John Wiley & Sons, 1977.

O'Regan, B. "Healing, Remission, and Miracle Cures." *Institute of Noetic Sciences Special Report* (May 1987): 3–14.

Ornstein, R. *On the Experience of Time.* London: Penguin Books, 1969.

Ornstein, R. *Psychology: The Study of Human Experience.* New York: Harcourt Brace Jovanovich, 1988.

Ornstein, R., and Sobel, D. *The Healing Brain: Breakthrough Discoveries About How the Brain Keeps Us Healthy.* New York: Simon & Schuster, 1987.

Ottewell, G. *The Thousand-Yard Model.* Greenville, SC: Furman University Press, 1989.

Owen, R. *Qualitative Research: The Early Years.* Salem, OR: Grayhaven Books, 1988.

Pearsall, P. *Super Immunity: Master Your Emotions and Improve Your Health.* New York: McGraw-Hill, 1987.

Pearsall, Paul. *Super Marital Sex: Loving for Life.* New York: Doubleday, 1989.

Peat, D. *Synchronicity: The Bridge Between Matter and Mind.* New York: Bantam Books, 1988.

Peck, S. *The Road Less Traveled.* New York: Simon & Schuster, 1976.

Pehek, J. O., Kyler, H. J., and Faust, D. L. "Image Modulations in Corona Discharge Photography." *Science* 15 (1976): 263–270.

Penfield, W. *The Mystery of the Mind.* Princeton, NJ: Princeton University Press, 1975.

Penrose, R. *The Emperor's New Mind: Concerning Computers, Minds, and the Laws of Physics.* New York: Oxford University Press, 1989.

Perls, F. *Gestalt Therapy Verbatim*. New York: Bantam Books, 1969.

Pfleegor, R. O., and Mandel, L. "Interference of Independent Photon Beams." *Physical Review* 159, no. 5 (1967): 125–134.

Pickover, C. A. *Computers, Pattern, Chaos, and Beauty: Graphics from an Unseen World*. New York: St. Martin's Press, 1990.

Plato. *The Collected Dialogues*, ed. Edith Hamilton and Huntington Cairns. Bolingen Series no. LXXI, New York: Pantheon Books, 1961.

Popp, F. A. "Physical Aspects of Biophotons." *Experiences* 44 (1977).

Prat, S., and Schlemmer, J. "Electrophotography." *Journal of the Biological Photography Association* 7, no. 4 (1939): 145–148.

Prince, W. F. *The Enchanted Boundary*. Boston: Boston Society for Psychical Research, 1930.

Priestly, J. B. *Man and Time*. London: Aldus Books, 1964.

Regis, E. *Who Got Einstein's Office? Eccentricity and Genius at the Institute for Advanced Study*. New York: Addison-Wesley Publishing Company, Inc., 1987.

Sabom, M. *Recollections of Death*. London: Corgi, 1982.

Sanderson, I. "Editorial: A Fifth Force." *Pursuit* 5, no. 4 (1972).

Schrödinger, E. *What Is Life? and Mind and Matter*. London: Cambridge University Press, 1969.

Schrödinger, E. *My View of the World*. Woodbridge, CT: Ox Bow Press, 1983.

Schul, B. *The Psychic Power of Animals*. New York: Fawcett, 1977.

Sengtsan. *Verses on the Faith Mind*, trans. E. R. Clark. Sharon Springs, NY: Zen Center, 1975.

Sergeant, C., and Eysenck, H. *Explaining the Unexplained*. London: Weidenfeld and Nicolson, 1982.

Sheldrake. R. *A New Science of Life*. Los Angeles: J. P. Tarcher, 1981.

Sheldrake, R. *The Presence of the Past*. New York: Random House, 1981.

Singer, B. "To Believe or Not to Believe," in *Science and the Paranormal*, ed. G. O. Abell and B. Singer. New York: Charles Scribner's Sons, 1981.

Siskin, B., and Staller, J. *What Are the Chances? Risks, Odds, and Likelihood in Everyday Life*. New York: Crown Publishers, 1989.

Skinner, B. F. "The Force of Coincidence." *The Humanist* 37, no. 3 (1977).

Skinner, B. F. "Can Psychology Be a Science of Mind." *American Psychologist* 45, no. 11 (1990): 1206–1211.

Spinoza, B. *The Philosophy of Spinoza*, intro. Joseph Ratner. New York: Random House, 1927.

Spinoza, B. "Tractatus Theologico." *Politicus*, vol. 2.

Stevens, W. "New Eye on Nature: The Real Constant Is Eternal Turmoil." *New York Times*, July 31, 1990, pp. C1–C2.

Stevenson, I. "Research into the Evidence of Man's Survival After Death." *Journal of Nervous and Mental Disease* 165, no. 3 (1977).

Stuart, C. I. J. M. "Mixed Brain Dynamics: Neural Memory as a Macroscopic Ordered State." *Foundations of Physics* 9, nos. 3 and 4 (1979).

Swinburne, R. *The Concept of Miracle*. New York: Macmillan, 1970.

Targ, R., and Harary, K. *The Mind Race: Understanding and Using Psychic Abilities*. New York: Ballantine Books, 1984.

Targ, R., and Puthoof. *Mind Reach: Scientists Look at Psychic Ability*. New York: Dell Publishing, 1977.

Tart, C. *Waking Up: Overcoming the Obstacles to Human Potential*. Boston: Shambhala, 1987.

Thompson, W. I. *Evil and World Order*. New York: Harper & Row, 1976.

Tiller, W. "Present Scientific Understanding of the Kirlian Discharge Process." *Psychoenergetic Systems* 3, nos. 1–4 (1979).

Toynbee, A., and Koestler, A., eds. *Life After Death*. London: Weldenfeld and Nicolson, 1976.

Vaughan, A. *Incredible Coincidence*. Philadelphia: J. B. Lippincott, 1979.

von Franz, M. *On Divination and Synchronicity*. Toronto: Inner City Books, 1980.

Wagar, W. Warren. *A Short History of the Future*. Chicago: University of Chicago Press, 1989.

Wald, R. M. "Correlations and Causality in Quantum Field Theory" in *Quantum Concepts in Space and Time*, ed. R. Penrose and C. J. Isham. Oxford, UK: Oxford University Press, 1986.

Walsh, R. "The Psychologies of East and West: Contrasting Views of the Human Condition and Potential." *Beyond Health and Normality: Explorations of Exceptional Psychological Well-Being*, ed. R. Walsh and D. Shapiro. New York: Van Nostrand Reinhold, 1983.

Watson, L. *Lifetide: The Biology of Consciousness*. New York: Simon & Schuster, 1980.

Watson, L. *Gifts of Unknown Things*. New York: Simon & Schuster, 1986.

Weinberg, S. *The First Three Minutes*. New York: Basic Books, 1976.

Wheeler, D. R. *Journey to the Other Side*. New York: Ace Books, 1976.

Wheeler, J. "Genesis and Observership," in *Foundational Problems in the Special Sciences*. New York: Reidel, 1977.

Wheeler, J. "Beyond the Black Hole," in *Some Strangeness in the Proportion*, ed. H. Wolf. Reading, MA: Addison-Wesley Publishers, 1980.

White, J. *The Meeting of Science and Spirit: The Next Dynamic Stage of Human Evolution and How We Will Attain It*. New York: Paragon House, 1990.

Wilbur, K., ed. *Quantum Questions: Mystical Writings of the World's Great Physicists*. Boston: New Science Library, 1984.

Wilczek, F., and Devine, B. *Longing for the Harmonies: Themes and Variations from Modern Physics*. New York: W. W. Norton, 1987.

Williams, H. *Sacred Elephant*. New York: Crown Publishers, 1989.

Wolinsky, H. "Prayers Do Aid Sick, Study Finds." *Chicago Sun Times*, Jan. 26, 1986.

Zohar, D. *The Quantum Self: Human Nature and Consciousness Defined by the New Physics*. New York: William Morrow, 1990.

INDEX